MCQs for the MRCPCH Part 1

Other Examination Preparation Books Published by Petroc Press:

Padmanabhan Ramnarayan is the author of *Ram's MRCPCH Teaching* (*see* www.ramsteaching.com)

MCQs for the MRCPCH Part 1

Padmanabhan Ramnarayan, MBBS, MRCP (UK), MRCPCH

Specialist Registrar in Paediatrics
Paediatric Intensive Care Unit
St Mary's Hospital, Paddington, London W2 1NY, UK

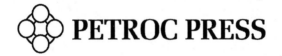 PETROC PRESS

Petroc Press, an imprint of LibraPharm Limited

Distributors
Plymbridge Distributors Limited, Plymbridge House, Estover Road, Plymouth
PL6 7PZ, UK

First edition 2002 © LibraPharm Limited

Published by LibraPharm Limited
Gemini House
162 Craven Road
Newbury
Berkshire
RG14 5NR
UK

A catalogue record for this book is available from the British Library

ISBN 1 900603 14 4

Typeset by Richard Powell Editorial and Production Services, Basingstoke,
Hampshire RG22 4TX

Printed and bound in the United Kingdom by AlphaGraphics, Preston Farm,
Stockton-on-Tees, TS18 3TR

Contents

Preface vii
Abbreviations ix

Questions 1

Section 1 3
Section 2 10
Section 3 17
Section 4 24
Section 5 31
Section 6 38
Section 7 45
Section 8 52
Section 9 59
Section 10 66

Answers 73

Section 1 75
Section 2 81
Section 3 88
Section 4 93
Section 5 99
Section 6 104
Section 7 111
Section 8 117
Section 9 123
Section 10 128

Scoring Sheets 135

Preface

Multiple choice questions are now a standard component of examinations in medicine. Most postgraduate examinations like the MRCP (UK) and the MRCS, as well as other examinations conducted abroad, use multiple choice questions to test examinees' knowledge of basic sciences and its application to practical real life clinical scenarios. The MRCPCH is no exception. This book is intended to assist paediatricians everywhere in their preparation for the MRCPCH examination.

All the questions in this book have been based (with modifications) from the popular *Ram's MRCPCH Teaching* website, which has had over 40,000 hits to date. I developed this resource over the past few years to assist trainees taking the MRCPCH examination in the UK and abroad. For the purpose of this book, however, all answers have been extensively revised and extended to cover more of the subject. Wherever possible, references have been added to assist further reading. Some of the choices within the questions have also been modified to reflect changes in the pattern of the examination over the last few years.

The questions themselves are not grouped by subject or by topic. Instead, I have set the questions in the form of 10 papers, each composed of 30 questions, to mirror the format of the examination, where each question consists of an initial stem followed by five items identified by A, B, C, D and E. There is no restriction on the number of true or false items in a question. It is possible for all the items in a question to be true, or for all to be false. Each item is independent of the others. The actual Part I examination is designed to assess a candidate's knowledge and understanding of the basic clinical sciences relevant to medical practice and of the common or important disorders to a level appropriate for the entry to higher specialist training. Questions may be set on the relevant principles of cell, molecular and membrane biology, on immunology, on genetics and on biochemistry, as well as on anatomical, physiological, microbiological and pharmacological topics.

Candidates indicate their answers to the questions by completing an answer sheet, which is machine-read by an optical mark reader (OMR). The output from the OMR is processed by computer. The computer allocates marks according to the candidates' responses, calculates their scores and derives statistical data relating to individual questions, and then produces this information in printed form for the examiners. To this end, Answers have been provided at the back, and scoring sheets have been added in order to facilitate the simulation of examination conditions. Much effort has gone into ensuring that all specialties and topics relevant to the MRCPCH have been covered within the framework of the sections. It has also been an arduous task to compose each of the questions and answers while continuing clinical duties, and I hope that the readers will appreciate the breadth of coverage and agree with most of the answers provided.

Finally, I hope that readers will find that this book does not completely satisfy their eagerness to learn and stimulates further reading on the topics covered. I express my gratitude to the thousands of users of my website, who have contributed in small and large measures to make the publication of this book possible. I hope they find this book more detailed, and in many ways, more complete, than the website itself.

London, June 2002   P.R.

Abbreviations

The following is a list of the abbreviations used throughout the text, together with their meanings:

ACE	Angiotensin converting enzyme	MELAS	Mitochondrial myopathy, encephalopathy, lactic acidosis and stroke-like episodes
AD	Autosomal dominant		
ALL	Acute lymphoblastic leukemia		
ANA	Anti-nuclear antibody	MERRF	Myoclonic epilepsy with ragged red fibres
AR	Autosomal recessive		
BPD	Bronchopulmonary dysplasia	NEC	Necrotising enterocolitis
CAH	Congenital adrenal hyperplasia	NF	Neurofibromatosis
		PEEP	Positive end-expiratory pressure
CDC	Communicable Diseases Center, Atlanta, GA, USA		
		PIP	peak inspiratory pressure
DDI	Didanosine	RDS	Respiratory distress syndrome
DKA	Diabetic ketoacidosis	RSV	Respiratory syncitial virus
DMSA	Dimercaptosuccinic acid	SCID	Severe combined immunodeficiency
EDS	Ehlers-Danlos syndrome		
EHBA	Extrahepatic biliary atresia	SVC	Superior vena cava
FFP	Fresh frozen plasma	SVT	Supraventricular tachycardia
GHRH	Growth hormone releasing hormone	TAPVD	Total anomalous pulmonary venous drainage
IGF	Insulin-like growth factor	TGA	Transposition of great arteries
INR	International normalised ratio	TOF	Tetralogy of Fallot
IVC	Inferior vena cava	URTIs	Upper respiratory tract infections
LFT	Liver function test		
MAP	Mean airway pressure	VIPoma	Vaso-active intestinal peptide
MCUG	Micturating cystourethrogram	VSD	Ventricular septal defect

Questions

Section 1

1.1   Regarding fluid and electrolyte homeostasis in a child:

(a) Normal maintenance requirement in a child weighing 20 kg is 1.5 litre/day
(b) A fluid deficit of 50 ml/kg produces a body weight loss of 10%
(c) Hypotension is a useful sign, which indicates moderate dehydration
(d) Normal maintenance needs of sodium are 5–6 mmol/kg/day
(e) The characteristic metabolic abnormality in a child with pyloric stenosis is hyperkalaemic hypochloraemic metabolic alkalosis

1.2   Sequelae of a complete posterior cord section between C3 and T1 include:

(a) Muscle fasciculation
(b) Loss of sensation below the lesion
(c) Loss of deep tendon reflexes
(d) Athetoid movements
(e) Sympathetic pseudomotor problems

1.3   The following conditions are associated with hyperammon-aemia:

(a) Reye syndrome
(b) Citrullinaemia
(c) Methylmalonic acidaemia
(d) Homocystinuria
(e) Isovaleric acidaemia

1.4   Membranous glomerulonephritis:

(a) Is typically associated with immune complex deposition
(b) Presents with nephritic syndrome
(c) Is associated with highly selective proteinuria
(d) Deposits of IgG on the glomerular membrane
(e) Carries a worse prognosis than minimal change disease

1.5 Common causes of jaundice in a 12-hour-old neonate include:

(a) Glucose-6-phosphate dehydrogenase deficiency
(b) Rhesus isoimmunisation
(c) Crigler–Najjar syndrome type II
(d) Choledochal cyst
(e) Breast-milk jaundice

1.6 Urinary tract infection:

(a) Usually leads to vesico-ureteric reflux
(b) Is more common in boys than girls under a year of age
(c) In boys, is most commonly caused by *Proteus mirabilis*
(d) Is associated with constipation
(e) Prevention is best achieved by long-term amoxycillin

1.7 Liver failure in children:

(a) Is always chronic in nature
(b) Wilson's disease is a common cause
(c) Leads to failure to thrive
(d) One of the causes is Reye syndrome
(e) Can result from unrecognised extrahepatic biliary atresia

1.8 Usual indications for an exchange transfusion in a child with sickle cell disease include:

(a) Painful vaso-occlusive crisis
(b) Splenic sequestration crisis
(c) Acute chest syndrome
(d) Dactylitis
(e) Priapism

1.9 Complications of an infant of a diabetic mother include:

(a) Hypoglycaemia
(b) Hypocalcaemia
(c) Hyperinsulinaemia
(d) Jaundice
(e) Hypomagnesaemia

1.10 Concerning SLE:

(a) Antibodies against double standard RNA are a typical finding
(b) Haematoxylin bodies occur in areas of inflammation
(c) Usually progresses to renal failure within two years
(d) Alopecia is a recognised finding
(e) Psychosis is a recognised presentation

1.11 Rett syndrome is characterised by:

(a) Social withdrawal
(b) Self-mutilation
(c) Macrocephaly
(d) Wringing hand movements
(e) Seizures

1.12 The following contribute to the natural immunity transmitted in breast milk:

(a) Macrophages
(b) Natural killer cells
(c) Lysozyme
(d) Mast cells
(e) Secretory IgA

1.13 Clubbing is found in:

(a) Crohn's disease
(b) Bronchiectasis
(c) Rheumatic fever
(d) Infective endocarditis
(e) Tetralogy of Fallot

1.14 Guillain-Barré syndrome (GBS) is excluded by:

(a) A normal CSF
(b) The presence of autonomic neuropathy
(c) Distinct sensory level
(d) Ophthalmoplegia
(e) Wasting

1.15 Common causes of recurrent abdominal pain include:

(a) Gilbert syndrome
(b) Chronic constipation
(c) Functional cause
(d) Familial Mediterranean fever
(e) Gastric ulcer

1.16 A diagnosis of primary pulmonary hypertension of the newborn can be made if:

(a) Oxygen saturation in the hand is 80%, and in the foot 67%
(b) A tachypnoeic baby has a saturation of 60%
(c) A baby with history of being covered in thick meconium at birth has PaO_2 of 4 kPa
(d) A septic baby is hypoxic in 100% oxygen
(e) The chest radiograph of a neonate with saturation of 40% shows a normal heart size

1.17 About juvenile chronic arthritis:

(a) Rheumatoid factor is an important diagnostic test to perform in suspected cases
(b) Pauciarticular type is the commonest type
(c) Cervical spine involvement is uncommon
(d) Methotrexate is the first line drug in therapy
(e) Extent of elevation of ESR at presentation is an important indicator of subsequent development of chronic iridocyclitis

1.18 Causes of pancytopenia and splenomegaly include:

(a) Low-grade non-Hodgkin's lymphoma
(b) Gaucher's disease
(c) Alcoholic cirrhosis
(d) B_{12} deficiency
(e) Aplastic anaemia

1.19 The following antibiotics interfere with bacterial translation:

(a) Penicillin
(b) Ceftriaxone
(c) Azithromycin
(d) Ciprofloxacin
(e) Sulphadiazine

1.20 Evidence of increased pulmonary flow is associated with:

(a) Coarctation of the aorta
(b) Fallot's tetralogy
(c) *Pneumocystis* infection
(d) Ventricular septal defect
(e) Eisenmenger's syndrome

1.21 Clinical manifestations of haemophilia include:

(a) Bleeding following neonatal intramuscular injection
(b) Intracranial bleeding
(c) Gingival bleeding
(d) Menorrhagia
(e) Bleeding following circumcision

1.22 Specific receptor defects occur in:

(a) Guillain–Barré syndrome
(b) Myasthenia gravis
(c) Graves' disease
(d) Ulcerative colitis
(e) Thyrotoxic exophthalmos

1.23 Possible causes of isosexual precocious puberty in a 6-year-old girl are:

(a) McCune–Albright syndrome
(b) Congenital adrenal hyperplasia (CAH)
(c) Ovarian tumour
(d) Hypothalamic hamartomas
(e) Constitutional cause

1.24   The following conditions may present with microcephaly:

(a) Dandy–Walker malformation
(b) Congenital rubella
(c) Rett syndrome
(d) Edward's syndrome
(e) Soto syndrome

1.25   The causes of elevated maternal serum AFP are:

(a) Trisomy 21
(b) Exomphalos
(c) Marfan syndrome
(d) Meningomyelocele
(e) Congenital nephrosis

1.26   Distal renal tubular acidosis:

(a) Is characterised by hypokalaemia
(b) May be primary or secondary
(c) Presents with growth failure in infancy
(d) Urinary pH is usually < 5
(e) Medullary nephrocalcinosis is a frequent finding

1.27   A seizure episode may be mimicked by:

(a) Breath-holding episode
(b) Choreoathetosis
(c) Hysterical reactions
(d) Vasovagal attack
(e) Benign paroxysmal vertigo

1.28   Appropriate investigations in the emergency management of a 4-year-old presenting in a coma:

(a) Serum magnesium level
(b) Throat swabs
(c) Arterial blood gas
(d) CT scan
(e) Blood cultures

1.29   Hyperkalaemia:

(a) Is exacerbated by acidosis
(b) Is a finding in Conn's syndrome
(c) ECG findings include peaked tall T-waves
(d) Should be treated if serum K_a > 6 mmol/l
(e) Insulin may be used in the management

1.30   Complications of long-term TPN administration are:

(a) Selenium deficiency
(b) Abnormal liver function tests
(c) Osteopaenia
(d) Renal failure
(e) Hyperglycaemia

Section 2

2.1 Regarding insulin administration in diabetics:

(a) Short-acting insulin reaches peak action in 4–6 hours after injection
(b) In a twice daily regimen involving Mixtard 30 or Humulin M3, the bedtime reading is an effect of the long-acting component
(c) A bedtime blood sugar level of 10 mmol/l is unacceptable
(d) Using the same site for injections is a common cause of increasing insulin dosage
(e) HbA1c levels are indicative of blood glucose levels in the past 12 weeks

2.2 True statements about the use of the new Child Health Foundation growth charts include:

(a) Immediate referral is advised if the height of a child is on the second centile
(b) The midparental height of a child, whose parents are 176 and 160 cm tall, is 175 cm
(c) They can be used for all children including those with Down's syndrome
(d) The target centile range for a girl is midparental height ± 10 cm
(e) The recording of head circumference is mandatory until a child is two years old

2.3 Tests used in establishing a diagnosis of coeliac disease are:

(a) IgA anti-endomysial antibodies
(b) IgM anti-reticulin antibodies
(c) IgA anti-gliadin antibodies
(d) Duodenal biopsy
(e) 72-hour faecal fat estimation

2.4 A child can be diagnosed as having Kawasaki disease if he has:

(a) Fever > 3 days' duration, > 38°C
(b) Purulent conjunctivitis
(c) Thrombocytosis
(d) Polymorphous rash
(e) Red tonsillar enlargement

2.5 Generalised absence seizures:

(a) Are usually atypical in type
(b) CT scan shows abnormalities in around 25–30% of cases
(c) Can be diagnosed in the absence of a typical EEG pattern with great certainty
(d) Are associated with other generalised seizures in most cases
(e) The typical EEG shows hypsarrythmia

2.6 Diseases that primarily involve the motor unit include:

(a) Werdnig–Hoffman disease
(b) Guillain–Barré syndrome
(c) Facioscapulohumeral dystrophy
(d) Tertiary syphilis
(e) Charcot–Marie–Tooth disease

2.7 Regarding café-au-lait spots:

(a) They can be normal findings
(b) They are found in tuberous sclerosis
(c) When present in a child, > 4 spots each > 0.5 cm, is diagnostic of neurofibromatosis type II
(d) Typical appearance in neurofibromatosis is of a smooth border
(e) They are found in most girls with precocious puberty

2.8 Polycythaemia:

(a) Is a common cause of jaundice in the newborn
(b) Is significant if haematocrit > 65% on a capillary sample
(c) May cause apnoeas
(d) Exchange transfusion is the treatment of choice in symptomatic cases
(e) Cerebellar haemangiomas are associated with it

2.9 The following conditions involve the oral mucosa:

(a) Herpes simplex type I infection
(b) Scabies
(c) Eczema
(d) Lichen planus
(e) Dermatitis herpetiformis

2.10 Appropriate initial management steps in an acute anaphylactic reaction to a blood transfusion include:

(a) Nebulised steroids
(b) Oxygen
(c) Intravenous hydrocortisone
(d) Intravenous anti-H_2 agent
(e) Accurate urine output measurement

2.11 Causes of hypertension in a child include:

(a) Long-standing vesico-ureteric reflux
(b) Cushing's syndrome
(c) Addison's disease
(d) 21-hydroxylase deficiency
(e) Turner's syndrome

2.12 Croup:

(a) Is a disease
(b) Is commonly caused by parainfluenza viruses
(c) Most cases are managed with nebulised adrenaline
(d) Inhaled steroids are reported to be of benefit
(e) Long-term complications are usually related to the duration of symptoms

2.13 Paediatric HIV infection:

(a) Is similar to adult HIV infection except for the mode of transmission
(b) Antenatal screening of pregnant women is not of proven benefit
(c) Developmental delay is a recognised presentation
(d) In an infant, the diagnosis is established first before any management steps are undertaken
(e) Most cases are due to transmission after birth, rather than transplacental

2.14 The following statements are true about screening:

(a) The sensitivity of a screening test is the extent of picking up true negatives
(b) Positive predictive value is dependent on the population being screened
(c) A good screening test is always inexpensive
(d) Screening for Duchenne muscular dystrophy is not practised, mainly because of the extent of false positives in the test
(e) A specificity value of > 80% is acceptable in a screening test

2.15 Possible causes of upper airway obstruction are:

(a) Inhaled foreign body in the main bronchus on the right side
(b) Epiglottitis
(c) Retropharyngeal abscess
(d) Bronchiolitis
(e) Viral croup

2.16 Nystagmus can be a presenting sign in:

(a) Partial albinism
(b) Retinopathy of prematurity
(c) Acute vestibulitis
(d) Medulloblastoma
(e) Phenytoin toxicity

2.17 Routine hearing tests in the community are usually based on:

(a) Distraction testing
(b) Auditory brainstem responses
(c) Evoked potentials
(d) Object discrimination
(e) Auditory cradle

2.18 Which of the following children are abnormal?

(a) 18-month-old who is able to put three blocks on top of each other and has a 2-word vocabulary
(b) 3-month-old who has just attained good head control, and is reaching for objects
(c) 5-year-old with difficulty in reading sentences from a book
(d) Bottom-shuffler who is still not walking at 16 months
(e) A 12-month-old boy who waves goodbye, and has a two-word vocabulary

2.19 Regarding puberty:

(a) The beginning of puberty is closely related to bony changes rather than to age
(b) The first sign of puberty in a boy is the development of axillary hair
(c) Constitutional precocious puberty is commoner in girls than boys
(d) Delayed puberty is defined as lack of pubertal changes in a boy after 14 years of age
(e) 21-hydroxylase deficiency is a cause of precocious puberty in boys

2.20   Complement system:

(a) Is activated by bacterial endotoxins by the classical pathway
(b) Reduced C3 and C4 are usual findings in acute glomerulonephritis
(c) Hereditary angioneurotic oedema is caused by deficiency of one of the components of the classical pathway of the system
(d) Is part of humoral immunity
(e) The final products of the classical pathway act by causing cell lysis

2.21   Diagnostic signs of child abuse are:

(a) Sub-hyaloid bleeding
(b) Spiral fracture of a long bone
(c) Lacerated tongue
(d) Posterior rib fractures
(e) Persistent vaginal discharge

2.22   The routine investigation of a 4-year-old with an uncomplicated UTI involves:

(a) Renal ultrasound scan
(b) Micturating cystogram
(c) DMSA (dimercaptosuccinic acid) scan
(d) DTP scan
(e) Intravenous urogram

2.23   The following drugs induce hepatic enzymes:

(a) Rifampicin
(b) Phenobarbitone
(c) Cimetidine
(d) Erythromycin
(e) Sodium valproate

2.24   Regarding hypogonadotropic hypogonadism:

(a) Kallman syndrome is an example
(b) It is caused by testicular atrophy secondary to trauma
(c) LHRH testing is used to distinguish it from other forms of hypogonadism
(d) It is treated with buserelin sprays
(e) It leads to obesity and micropenis

2.25 Prader Willi syndrome:

(a) Is caused by a maternal deletion of a part of chromosome 15
(b) Presents with macrosomia in infancy
(c) Developmental delay is common
(d) Behavioural problems are common
(e) Results in excessive feeding in infants

2.26 Childhood autism:

(a) Is commoner in boys
(b) Is characterised by extreme delay of social milestones
(c) Repetitive tasks are commonly performed
(d) Is characterised by extremely chaotic routines
(e) Has a good prognosis

2.27 The following diseases have diagnostic EEG findings:

(a) Petit mal epilepsy
(b) Infantile spasms
(c) Acute measles encephalopathy
(d) Herpes encephalitis
(e) Tonic seizures

2.28 Causes of a dilated renal pelvis in a foetal scan include:

(a) Normal variant
(b) Vesico-ureteric reflux
(c) Pelvi-ureteric junction obstruction
(d) Multicystic kidney
(e) Neuroblastoma

2.29 Neural crest derivatives include:

(a) Adrenal cortical cells
(b) Melanocytes
(c) Langerhans cells
(d) Gastric epithelial cells
(e) Glial cells

2.30 Short stature due to growth hormone deficiency:

(a) Is characteristically manifest in infancy
(b) May be secondary to irradiation to the skull
(c) Can be part of congenital hypopituitarism
(d) Is easily corrected
(e) Is always associated with other hormonal deficiencies

Section 3

3.1 In childhood asthma:

(a) Over 90% of patients show exercise-induced bronchoconstriction
(b) Hypercapnia is the first physiological disturbance in status asthmaticus
(c) Infants are unresponsive to bronchodilators
(d) Spontaneous cure occurs before adolescence
(e) Cough may be the only symptom

3.2 The following statements concerning acute gastroenteritis in childhood are correct:

(a) Intravenous fluid therapy is essential in severe cases
(b) Loperamide should be avoided
(c) The commonest causes of failure to thrive following an attack is persistent bacterial infection
(d) Septicaemia is a recognised feature of *Salmonella* gastroenteritis
(e) Breast-feeding should be continued throughout the illness

3.3 The following conditions can present in a newborn infant as a bullous eruption:

(a) Syphilis
(b) Mast cell disease
(c) Epidermolysis bullosa
(d) Phenylketonuria
(e) Atopic eczema

3.4 A 4-year-old child has had fever, malaise, and vomiting and right-sided abdominal pain for 48 hours. The following are likely diagnoses:

(a) Acute pyelonephritis
(b) *Shigella* dysentery
(c) *Ascaris lumbricoides* infestation, if the child is living in the tropics
(d) Right sided tumour
(e) Lobar pneumonia

3.5 Recognised diagnoses of tender scrotal swelling in infancy include:

(a) Inguinal hernia
(b) Epididymo-orchitis
(c) Breech delivery
(d) Torsion of testis
(e) Orchidoblastoma

3.6 Which is/are true?

(a) Babies are able to respond to sounds *in utero*
(b) Full term babies at birth are unable to follow a large object with their eyes
(c) A 6-week-old infant would be able to follow a large object through an arc of 135°
(d) Growth velocity of head decreases with age
(e) A 12-month-old infant who keeps falling when starting to walk is likely to have cerebral palsy

3.7 The following statements regarding retinoblastoma are correct:

(a) It is usually fatal even if diagnosis is made early
(b) The tumour is heritable
(c) They may occur bilaterally
(d) The finding of leucorrhoea suggests the diagnosis
(e) It may present with heterochromia iris

3.8 A child aged 10 days has ambiguous genitalia:

(a) If a buccal smear is chromatin negative, there is a serious risk of an Addisonian crisis
(b) A raised urinary output of pregnanetriol would confirm a diagnosis of CAH
(c) The finding of the genotype 45 XO would reliably explain the anomaly
(d) If testicles were present in the 'labia', an acceptable explanation would be Klinefelter's syndrome
(e) The most important factor in deciding the sex to which the child should be assigned is the genetic (chromosomal) sex

3.9 In infantile eczema:

(a) The rash is characteristically present at birth
(b) The papules are itchy
(c) Cold weather relieves the symptoms
(d) A family history of related disorders is elicited in 70% of cases
(e) Dermographism excludes the diagnosis

3.10 Obesity in childhood:

(a) Is usually associated with hypogonadism
(b) Is unlikely to lead to adult obesity
(c) Is more common in families in Social Class I than in Social Class V
(d) Can lead to overestimation of the dose of intravenous fluids when these are required
(e) Is usually associated with above average height before puberty

3.11 A 2-year-old child should be able to:

(a) Name three colours correctly
(b) Use plurals
(c) Build a tower of five blocks
(d) Kick a ball on request
(e) Hop on one foot

3.12 Acute bronchiolitis is associated with:

(a) A higher incidence in infants than in school children
(b) The production of copious amounts of purulent sputum
(c) Widespread fine crackles
(d) A polymorphonuclear leucocytosis
(e) Respiratory syncitial virus infection

3.13 Which of the following skills would be expected of a 7-month-old infant but not of a 5-month-old infant?

(a) Crawls
(b) Smiles socially
(c) Controls bowel and bladder
(d) Sits unsupported
(e) Raises head while prone

3.14 In childhood, hypokalaemic alkalosis is a recognised finding:

(a) In a baby given feeds that are too concentrated
(b) In congenital pyloric stenosis
(c) In cystic fibrosis
(d) Following urinary diversion
(e) In renal failure

3.15 Childhood schizophrenia is suggested by:

(a) Disturbance in movement patterns
(b) Persistent thumb sucking
(c) Hallucinations
(d) Infantile autism
(e) Negativism

3.16 Progressive spinal muscular atrophy of infancy presents with:

(a) Severe generalised weakness
(b) Fasciculations in the tongue
(c) Loss of spinothalamic tract function
(d) Spontaneous fibrillation on electromyography
(e) Normal tendon reflexes

3.17 Psychosis in children is suggested by:

(a) Absence of speech
(b) Intense outbursts of temper
(c) Recurrence of bed-wetting following a period of control
(d) Feelings of depersonalisation
(e) Sudden onset of stuttering

3.18 Inability to do which of the following in a 20-month child is cause for concern?

(a) Speak in clear two to three word phrases
(b) Walk unaided
(c) Kick a ball
(d) Build a tower of 8 blocks
(e) Co-operate with dressing

3.19 The following statements are true of bronchiolitis:

(a) Up to 50% of patients continue to wheeze after recovery
(b) The typical pathogen is para-influenza virus
(c) Corticosteroid therapy is beneficial
(d) Tachypnoea is invariable
(e) Air-trapping is normally present

3.20 An infant aged 16 months was referred for assessment of suspected mental retardation. Which of the following findings is/are outside the normal range?

(a) He does not scribble spontaneously with pencil on paper
(b) He does not walk alone
(c) 'Ma' and 'Dada' are the only recognisable words
(d) He is unable to build a tower of four cubes
(e) He is unable to throw an object

3.21 The pH of urine:

(a) Is a useful indicator of the acid/base balance of blood
(b) Rises on a vegetarian diet
(c) Is determined by the concentration of ammonium
(d) Is lower than 5.5 in renal tubular acidosis
(e) Would be above 7.0 after prolonged and severe vomiting

3.22 The following drugs cause hypokalaemia:

(a) Commencement of digoxin for atrial fibrillation
(b) ACE (angiotensin converting enzyme) inhibitors
(c) Salbutamol for asthma
(d) Vitamin B_{12} for the treatment of pernicious anaemia
(e) Cimetidine for duodenal ulcer

3.23 Avascular necrosis of the femoral head is associated with:

(a) Sickle cell trait
(b) Nephrotic syndrome
(c) Cushing's syndrome
(d) Hypothyroidism
(e) Gaucher's disease

3.24 The following are features of encephalitis:

(a) Herpes simplex encephalitis has a reasonably good prognosis
(b) Varicella zoster virus encephalitis is predominantly 'cerebellar'
(c) Mumps encephalitis can cause unilateral nerve deafness
(d) Herpes simplex encephalitis predominantly affects the temporal lobe
(e) Herpes simplex encephalitis causes a blood stained CSF

3.25 Renal damage is a recognised complication of infection with:

(a) *Plasmodium falciparum*
(b) *Schistosoma haematobium*
(c) *Plasmodium malariae*
(d) *Leptospira icterohaemorrhagica*
(e) *Mycobacterium leprae*

3.26 Abnormal coloration of the urine (in the absence of haematuria) may be due to:

(a) Consumption of beetroot
(b) Treatment with co-danthramer
(c) Phenylketonuria
(d) Acute intermittent porphyria
(e) Acute intravascular haemolysis

3.27 The following cranial nerves carry pre-ganglionic parasympathetic nerves:

(a) Oculomotor nerve
(b) Trigeminal nerve
(c) Facial nerve
(d) Vagus nerve
(e) Trochlear (IV) nerve

3.28 The following are recognised features of achondroplasia:

(a) Shortened spine
(b) Increased liability to pathological fractures
(c) Can be diagnosed radiologically at birth
(d) Infertility
(e) Autosomal recessive inheritance

3.29 Azathioprine:

(a) Is a prodrug
(b) Is teratogenic
(c) Should be avoided in liver disease
(d) Dose should be increased when given with allopurinol
(e) Is a recognised cause of pancreatitis

3.30 Distal occlusion of the posterior cerebral artery may produce:

(a) Contralateral hemiplegia
(b) Homonymous hemianopia
(c) Dysarthria
(d) Cerebellar ataxia
(e) Palatal palsy

Section 4

4.1 Features predisposing to NEC (necrotising enterocolitis) in the neonatal period include:

(a) Short fixation
(b) Asphyxia
(c) Umbilical artery catheter
(d) Maternal Crohn's disease
(e) Hirschsprung's disease

4.2 Typical features of Down's syndrome include:

(a) Brachycephaly
(b) Polydactyly
(c) Male infertility
(d) Increased α-fetoprotein in amniotic fluid
(e) Hypotonia

4.3 The following drugs are contraindicated in renal failure:

(a) Nitrofurantoin
(b) Carbamazepine
(c) Salbutamol
(d) Metolazone
(e) Erythromycin

4.4 Bronchoconstriction is a recognised side effect of:

(a) Captopril
(b) Atenolol
(c) Ibuprofen
(d) Paracetamol
(e) Salbutamol

4.5 Type I renal tubular acidosis:

(a) Only occurs in children
(b) Is caused by a failure of ammonium ion secretion
(c) Is associated with renal calcification
(d) Typically leads to hypovolaemia
(e) Characteristically, there is a failure to acidify urine below pH 7

4.6 In the most common type of CAH:

(a) There is deficient 11-hydroxylase
(b) Hypertension is a feature
(c) There is an associated gene defect
(d) Transmission is autosomal dominant
(e) Plasma levels of 17-hydroxyprogesterone are increased

4.7 In bronchopulmonary dysplasia:

(a) Lung compliance is increased
(b) Bronchial reactivity is increased
(c) Lung function typically improves with age
(d) Hyperinflation is an associated finding
(e) Inhaled steroids are useful

4.8 The following are associated with an increased risk of fetal abnormalities:

(a) Oligohydramnios
(b) Maternal HIV
(c) Paternal diabetes
(d) Decreased α-fetoprotein level
(e) A previous sibling with anencephaly

4.9 Methaemoglobinaemia may occur as a result of ingestion or exposure to:

(a) Paraquat
(b) Methylene blue
(c) Potassium permanganate
(d) Nitrates
(e) Ascorbic acid

4.10 Duchenne muscular dystrophy:

(a) Has an association with malignant hyperpyrexia
(b) Is a reason for never running properly
(c) Is better diagnosed with muscle biopsy than gene probe
(d) Is associated with speech delay
(e) Is a recognised cause of a floppy baby

4.11 In systemic mastocytosis:

(a) Areas of depigmentation occur
(b) Intermittent bronchoconstriction is characteristic
(c) IgE levels are high
(d) Is relieved by aspirin
(e) Intermittent flushing is seen

4.12 In Wolf–Parkinson–White syndrome:

(a) The abnormal pathway is between the atrial and ventricular myo-cardium
(b) Wide QRS complexes occur more frequently than narrow QRS
(c) Narrow QRS complexes are regular
(d) Verapamil is the treatment of choice for atrial fibrillation
(e) Amiodarone increases the refractory period of AV node

4.13 Early features of heart failure in infancy include:

(a) Bradycardia
(b) Oedema
(c) Tachypnoea
(d) Hepatomegaly
(e) Cyanosis

4.14 Congenital toxoplasmosis is associated with:

(a) Microcephaly
(b) Cervical lymphadenopathy
(c) Sore throat
(d) Sacroileitis
(e) Chorioretinitis

4.15   Consequences of a median nerve section in the ante-cubital fossa include:

(a) Complete paralysis of pronation
(b) Loss of sensation over palmar aspect of middle finger
(c) Wasting of hypothenar eminence
(d) Paralysis of abductor pollicis brevis
(e) Inability to extend ring finger

4.16   Causes of a discrete osteolytic bone lesion in a two-year old include:

(a) Rickets
(b) Non-accidental injury
(c) Eosinophilic granuloma
(d) Acute lymphoblastic leukaemia
(e) Bone cyst

4.17   Regarding body iron stores:

(a) Serum ferritin is a poor guide to iron stores
(b) A healthy young man will have more iron stored as ferritin than in the circulating red cell mass
(c) Iron is the stimulant for ferritin production
(d) In iron deficiency, stores of haemosiderin are mobilised before ferritin
(e) If stained with nitroprusside stain both haemosiderin and transferrin have the same colour

4.18   Petit mal epilepsy:

(a) Is the usual cause of drop attacks
(b) Demonstrates a specific EEG pattern
(c) More common pre- than post-pubertal
(d) Is likely to lead to poor school performance if not treated
(e) Is treated with clonazepam

4.19   The following are associated with cystic fibrosis:

(a) Nasal polyps
(b) Biliary cirrhosis
(c) Low sweat Na^+ content
(d) Chromosomal abnormality
(e) Bartter syndrome

4.20 Concerning sexual abuse in children:

(a) All abused children should be tested for HIV
(b) It is rare in children less than one year
(c) Girls are 20 times more likely to be abused than boys
(d) An abused child is likely to become a child abuser
(e) There are often few physical signs

4.21 Plethoric lung fields are seen in:

(a) *Pneumocystis carinii* infection
(b) Coarctation of aorta
(c) Large VSD (ventricular septal defect)
(d) Fallot's syndrome
(e) Eisenmenger's syndrome

4.22 Regarding gut hormones:

(a) Gastrin stimulates gastric motility
(b) Secretin is responsible for mucosal growth
(c) Enterokinase inhibits gastrin secretion
(d) Secretin is responsible for pancreatic bicarbonate secretion
(e) Somatostatin inhibits gastric secretion

4.23 Tumour necrosis factor:

(a) Is associated with an increase in appetite
(b) Is involved in rheumatoid arthritis
(c) Is released by mast cells
(d) Is increased in neurofibromatosis
(e) Indicates the presence of malignancy

4.24 Concerning RSV (respiratory syncitial virus) associated bronchiolitis:

(a) An effective vaccine is available
(b) Treatment of choice is aciclovir
(c) There is a high mortality in babies with congenital heart defects
(d) Disease can be prevented after contact by administration of high concentrate RSV immunoglobulin
(e) It can result in a post-bronchiolitic croupy stage

4.25 Recognised features of brucellosis include:

(a) Epididymo-orchitis
(b) Leucoplakia
(c) Vesicular eruption
(d) Positive Weil's test
(e) Recurrent fever

4.26 Toxin-mediated *Staphylococcus*:

(a) May cause diarrhoea and vomiting
(b) Can lead to toxic shock syndrome
(c) Is the cause of scalded skin syndrome
(d) Leads to peripheral neuropathy
(e) Works by acting as a superantigen

4.27 Standard deviation:

(a) Is the square of the variance
(b) Is a higher value than SEM
(c) Measures the scatter of data around the mean
(d) Is used to calculate the chi-square
(e) Can only be used in a normally distributed population

4.28 In Wilson's disease:

(a) There is an association with high caeruloplasmin levels
(b) Hepatic copper deposition is pathognomonic
(c) There is increased urinary excretion of copper
(d) There are copper deposits on the cornea
(e) Psychiatric manifestations are common

4.29 In protein energy malnutrition:

(a) Albumin is typically low
(b) RT3 levels are decreased
(c) There is increased reaction to tuberculin testing
(d) Fatty liver is a recognised finding
(e) Levels of IgE are increased

4.30 The following tests are routine in the management of an epileptic on carbamazepine:

(a) Blood counts
(b) Serum levels
(c) Liver function tests
(d) Renal function tests
(e) MRI scan

Section 5

5.1 Klinefelter's syndrome:

(a) Has a karyotype XXY
(b) Is the result of meiotic non-dysjunction
(c) Shows delay in bone age/maturation
(d) Is a recognised cause of hypogonadotrophic hypogonadism
(e) Is inherited as an X-linked recessive trait

5.2 Mental retardation is found in all the following:

(a) Trisomy 21
(b) Morquio syndrome
(c) Homocystinuria
(d) Ehlers–Danlos syndrome
(e) Cornelia de Lange syndrome

5.3 The following are transmitted as autosomal dominant traits:

(a) Congenital spherocytosis
(b) Vitamin D-resistant rickets
(c) CAH
(d) Hereditary haemorrhagic telangiectasia
(e) Wilson's disease

5.4 Dubowitz criteria to assess gestational age include:

(a) Skin colour
(b) Breast tissue
(c) Popliteal angle
(d) Moro reflex
(e) Scarf sign

5.5   Cataracts are recognised in:

(a) Hyperthyroidism
(b) Down syndrome
(c) Graves' disease
(d) PKU
(e) Toxoplasma

5.6 Chief organ systems affected in acute graft-versus-host reaction are:

(a) Skin
(b) Renal system
(c) Gut
(d) CNS
(e) Haematological

5.7   The following causes of short stature respond to growth hormone:

(a) Turner's syndrome
(b) Panhypopituitarism
(c) Achondroplasia
(d) Social deprivation
(e) Craniopharyngioma

5.8   Concerning insulin-dependent diabetes mellitus in children:

(a) Microangiopathic changes are rare before puberty
(b) Isophane is shorter acting than soluble insulin
(c) Lipohypertrophy is more common than lipo-atrophy
(d) Fructosamine can be used to monitor glucose control
(e) It is always part of an autoimmune syndrome

5.9   A pulmonary embolus occurring while the patient is on the combined oral contraceptive pill:

(a) Is more likely in anti-thrombin III deficiency
(b) Is more likely in protein C deficiency
(c) Is an absolute contraindication to the combined pill
(d) Is an increased risk in smokers
(e) The thrombotic tendency is due to the progesterone component

5.10 Emergency management of acute asthma includes:

(a) Arterial blood gas
(b) Nebulised steroids
(c) Intravenous theophylline
(d) Nebulised β-antagonists
(e) Intravenous hydrocortisone

5.11 Concerning bulimia nervosa:

(a) Review of teeth may aid diagnosis
(b) Patients may get hypokalaemia
(c) Patients are likely to neglect their appearance
(d) There is an association with calluses on the dorsum of hands
(e) Patients are likely to be underweight

5.12 Examples of cyanotic heart disease include:

(a) Ebstein's anomaly
(b) Pulmonary stenosis
(c) Coarctation of aorta
(d) Hypoplastic left heart syndrome
(e) Supradiaphragmatic TAPVD (total anomalous pulmonary venous drainage)

5.13 The following are causes of cyanosis in the presence of 60% oxygen:

(a) Haemoglobin concentration < 5 g%
(b) Methaemoglobinaemia
(c) Thalassaemia
(d) Right to left shunt
(e) Eisenmenger's syndrome

5.14 Treatment options in the management of an intusussception include:

(a) Contrast enema
(b) Air enema
(c) Water enema
(d) Open surgery
(e) Endoscopic reduction

5.15 Concerning Ebstein–Barr virus (infectious mononucleosis):

(a) Presence of petechiae between the hard and soft palate supports the diagnosis
(b) Typically a rash following administration of penicillin V occurs
(c) Guillain–Barré syndrome is a recognised sequel
(d) Hepatitis is common
(e) Cervical lymphadenopathy and splenomegaly are due to extreme B cell hyperactivity

5.16 A child of 36 months would be expected to:

(a) Build a tower of 5 cubes
(b) Repeat back 5 digits
(c) Draw a man with a head and body
(d) Demonstrate symbolic play
(e) Know 4 colours

5.17 Recognised causes of delayed speech include:

(a) Hypothyroidism
(b) PKU
(c) Cystinuria
(d) Twins
(e) Deafness

5.18 Coxsackie viruses are implicated in:

(a) Herpangina
(b) Dermatitis herpetiformis
(c) Meningitis
(d) Orchitis
(e) Epidemic pleurodynia

5.19 Features that would increase suspicion of cerebral palsy at age 9 months include:

(a) Presence of Moro reflex
(b) Abductor spasm
(c) Hand dominance
(d) Grasp reflex
(e) Extensor plantar reflexes

5.20 Extracorpuscular causes of haemolysis include:

(a) α-Thalassaemia
(b) Hereditary ovalocytosis
(c) Warm antibody autoimmune haemolytic anaemia
(d) Pyruvate kinase deficiency
(e) Hypersplenism

5.21 Prevalence of psychiatric disorder:

(a) Is higher in urban than in rural areas
(b) Is increased in children with moderate learning difficulties
(c) Is increased in severe physical disability
(d) Is higher in children in social service care
(e) Is increased in children adopted shortly after birth

5.22 Causes of a loin mass and haematuria:

(a) Wilm's tumour
(b) Polycystic kidney disease
(c) Pyonephrosis
(d) Renal vein thrombosis
(e) Haemolytic uraemic syndrome

5.23 The following favour a non-organic (psychological) cause of abdominal pain:

(a) Two-year history
(b) Family history of peptic ulcer
(c) Family history of migraine
(d) Absence from school
(e) Presence of mouth ulcers

5.24 Causes of non-bloody diarrhoea include:

(a) *Shigella* dysentery
(b) *Campylobacter jejuni*
(c) *Giardia lamblia*
(d) *Salmonella*
(e) Antibiotic associated colitis

5.25 Galactosaemia:

(a) Exhibits autosomal recessive inheritance
(b) Is associated with cataracts
(c) Results in a low glucose level
(d) Is due to an inability to convert galactose into glucose
(e) Causes a positive glucose oxidation test

5.26 *Mycoplasma* pneumonia:

(a) Is associated with bullous myringitis
(b) Cold haemaglutinin antibodies are a recognised finding
(c) Guillain–Barré syndrome is a recognised sequel
(d) Is associated with erythema marginatum
(e) Is associated with thrombocytopenic purpura

5.27 The following are true of umbilical hernia:

(a) It is more common in Caucasian than Blacks
(b) It is commonly associated with hypothyroidism
(c) It must be operated on by two years of age
(d) It becomes obstructed in 2% of cases
(e) It is more likely to resolve spontaneously if small

5.28 In embryology:

(a) Most defects occur with teratogens in the first 2 weeks post-conception
(b) The urachus becomes the median umbilical ligament
(c) The mesonephric duct becomes the male organs
(d) The thyroid develops from the floor of the primitive larynx
(e) Melanocytes originate from neural crest cells

5.29 Recognised features of ABO incompatibility include:

(a) Normal haemoglobin on day 1
(b) Worsening with subsequent pregnancies
(c) Conjugated hyperbilirubinaemia
(d) Negative Coombs test
(e) May occur in first pregnancy

5.30 The following are true of vitamin K:

(a) It is a water-soluble vitamin
(b) It is found mainly in red meat
(c) After infancy most is synthesised by the gut flora
(d) Levels may be low in biliary obstruction
(e) Low levels after birth may lead to intracerebral haemorrhage

Section 6

6.1 Regarding the genetics of CF:

(a) The commonest mutation in Caucasians is the ΔF-580
(b) Parents of the affected child will show some symptoms in childhood
(c) Accurate prenatal diagnosis is possible in all cases
(d) There are less than 10 mutations causing disease
(e) The affected protein is a transmembrane Na channel

6.2 Initial tests in a 2-year-old child with failure to thrive include:

(a) Thyroid function tests
(b) Jejunal biopsy
(c) Urine culture
(d) Colonoscopy
(e) Sweat test

6.3 Biochemical abnormalities in a chronic carrier of hepatitis B are:

(a) Raised AST
(b) Low serum albumin
(c) Raised gamma GT
(d) Raised transferrin
(e) Urinary bilirubin

6.4 Commonly used anti-epileptic drugs in children include:

(a) Sodium valproate
(b) Lamotrigine
(c) Topiramate
(d) Phenytoin
(e) Carbamazepine

6.5   Management of a patient with an INR (insulin-like growth factor) of 8.7 from warfarin overdose includes:

(a) Vitamin K
(b) Cryoprecipitate
(c) Fresh frozen plasma
(d) Desmopressin
(e) Tranexamic acid

6.6   The following investigations are not needed in a 3-year old on TPN for the past 3 weeks:

(a) Serum selenium
(b) Serum manganese
(c) Serum iron
(d) Serum calcium
(e) Serum phosphate

6.7   Causes of hypogonadotropic hypogonadism are:

(a) Kallman's syndrome
(b) Testicular atrophy
(c) Klinefelter's syndrome
(d) Hypothalamic tumour
(e) Prader Willi syndrome

6.8   Causes of short stature include:

(a) Steroids at a dose of > 2 mg/kg for 4 weeks
(b) Osteogenesis imperfecta
(c) Hypochondroplasia
(d) Morquio syndrome
(e) 11β-OH deficiency

6.9   Common causes of recurrent haematuria are:

(a) Berger's disease
(b) Goodpasture's syndrome
(c) Renal stones
(d) Acute post-streptococcal glomerulonephritis
(e) Alport's syndrome

6.10 The following drugs are given by subcutaneous route:

(a) Human GH
(b) Insulin
(c) Human erythropoietin
(d) Hepatitis B vaccine
(e) Desferrioxamine

6.11 Management of a thalassaemia includes:

(a) Whole blood transfusions
(b) Pneumovax
(c) Bone marrow transplant
(d) Penicillin V prophylaxis
(e) Desferrioxamine

6.12 Pulmonary hypertension is a complication of:

(a) ASD
(b) TOF (tetralogy of Fallot)
(c) Tricuspid atresia
(d) Tricuspid regurgitation
(e) Eisenmenger syndrome

6.13 Recurrent headaches in childhood are seen with:

(a) Tension headaches
(b) Migraine
(c) Sinusitis
(d) Hypermetropia
(e) Recurrent embolic phenomena in the cerebral vessels

6.14 Fetal distress is indicated by:

(a) Meconium staining of liquor
(b) Arrhythmias
(c) Tachycardia
(d) Bradycardia
(e) Type I decelerations

6.15 Common reasons for doing a BMT in children are:

(a) SCID (severe combined immunodeficiency)
(b) Acute lymphoblastic leukemia
(c) CML
(d) Gaucher's disease
(e) Aplastic anaemia

6.16 False statements include:

(a) Curosurf is a natural surfactant
(b) Antenatal steroids are usually given as two oral doses of dexamethasone
(c) Increasing the rate on the ventilator raises the mean airway pressure
(d) CPAP is a common weaning tool in ventilated preterms
(e) The pressure–volume curve of the lung shifts to the left with surfactant administration

6.17 Recognised associations of Addison's disease include:

(a) Neurofibromatosis
(b) Phaeochromocytoma
(c) IDDM
(d) Nephrogenic diabetes insipidus
(e) Hashimoto's thyroiditis

6.18 Uncommon complications of severe falciparum malaria are:

(a) Stroke
(b) Anaemia
(c) Hepatitis
(d) Jaundice
(e) Hypoglycaemia

6.19 Triggers of the alternate pathway of complement are:

(a) Bacterial lipopolysaccharide
(b) Interleukin 2
(c) Macrophages
(d) Properdin
(e) C1 esterase

6.20 These causes often cause secretory diarrhoea except:

(a) Lactose intolerance
(b) *E. coli* infection
(c) Congenital chloridorrhoea
(d) Blind loop syndrome
(e) Cystic fibrosis

6.21 Neurodegenerative diseases include the following:

(a) Niemann–Pick disease
(b) Metachromatic leukodystrophy
(c) Leigh's encephalopathy
(d) Canavan disease
(e) Reye syndrome

6.22 Respiratory distress at birth is mostly caused by:

(a) Diaphragmatic hernia
(b) Meconium aspiration
(c) RDS (respiratory distress syndrome)
(d) Pulmonary hypertension
(e) Tricuspid stenosis

6.23 Accepted maintenance treatment for chronic asthma includes the following:

(a) High-dose inhaled steroids and long-acting bronchodilators
(b) Montelucast
(c) Montelucast and inhaled steroids
(d) Long-acting β_2-agonists alone
(e) Oral steroids plus high-dose inhaled steroids plus long acting β_2-agonists

6.24 Common causes of seizures in a neonate are:

(a) Hypocalcaemia
(b) Hypoglycaemia
(c) Pyridoxine deficiency
(d) Hydrocephalus
(e) Asphyxia

6.25 Toddler's diarrhoea is characterised by:

(a) Onset over 18 months
(b) Failure to thrive
(c) Excessive consumption of cow's milk
(d) Undigested food particles in the stool
(e) Anaemia

6.26 A VII nerve injury at the exit from the stylomastoid foramen would explain all except:

(a) Loss of sensation over the vallecula
(b) Loss of taste over the anterior third of the tongue
(c) Increased responsiveness to loud noises
(d) Inability to open the ipsilateral eye
(e) Loss of sensation over the cheek on the same side

6.27 Common pathogens in the sputum of CF patients are:

(a) *Pseudomonas*
(b) *Staphylococcus epidermidis*
(c) *Staphylococcus aureus*
(d) *Burkholderia*
(e) *Haemophilus*

6.28 Examples of encapsulated organisms are all except:

(a) *Pseudomonas*
(b) *Proteus*
(c) *Pneumococci*
(d) *Salmonella*
(e) *Neisseria meningitidis*

6.29 It is reasonable to suspect child abuse in the following situations:

(a) 6-month old with a large scalp bruise
(b) 7-year-old girl who is found masturbating
(c) 2-year old with multiple bruises of different ages over the shins
(d) 3-month old with failure to thrive
(e) 3-year old who is refusing to stay with the child minder in the last couple of weeks

6.30 The differential in a 5-year old with a 2-week history of painful joints is all the following except:

(a) Viral polyarthritis
(b) Still's disease
(c) Lyme disease
(d) Rheumatic fever
(e) Rheumatoid arthritis

Section 7

7.1 In homocystinuria:

(a) Homocysteine accumulates just proximal to the enzyme defect
(b) Osteoporosis is a recognised feature
(c) Oral contraceptive pills with oestrogens are contraindicated
(d) Dislocation of lens is a feature
(e) Skeletal features similar to Marfan's syndrome are seen

7.2 Coarctation of aorta is:

(a) Commonly associated with Turner's syndrome
(b) Inherited as autosomal dominant
(c) Associated with intracranial aneurysms
(d) Excluded from the diagnosis in the presence of femoral pulses
(e) Commonest congenital heart lesion seen

7.3 Regarding cough receptors:

(a) There is increased sensitivity in viral infections
(b) β_2-agonists decrease the sensitivity of cough receptors
(c) Exercise can stimulate the cough receptors in asthmatics
(d) They are predominantly seen in the large airways
(e) Codeine acts on the cough receptors to suppress cough

7.4 Regarding bronchial asthma:

(a) Mortality has shown an increase during the past three decades
(b) The incidence is greater in males than females
(c) Nocturnal cough is a recognised feature
(d) Post-RSV bronchial hyperreactivity is strongly associated with atopy
(e) Chronic asthma may decrease bone age by one year in an 8-year old

7.5 Drugs to be avoided in renal failure include:

(a) Allopurinol
(b) Rifampicin
(c) Ceftazidime
(d) Acyclovir
(e) Digoxin

7.6 Regarding hand innervation:

(a) Median nerve supplies all thenar muscles except adductor pollicis
(b) The sensory supply to the dorsal surface of the medial two digits is via the radial nerve
(c) In ulnar nerve damage at the elbow there is sensory loss over the medial aspect of forearm proximal to the wrist
(d) Radial nerve provides the sensory innervation to the terminal areas of the dorsal surfaces of the lateral three digits
(e) Dorsal interossei are supplied by the radial nerve

7.7 Regarding cranial nerves:

(a) Meningioma of the olfactory groove may cause unilateral anosmia
(b) Lesion in the geniculate ganglion produces hyperacusis
(c) Frontalis muscle is spared in lower motor neuron facial palsy
(d) In oculomotor palsy, pupillary sparing occurs in early stages of external compression of the nerve by a tumour
(e) Occlusion of internal auditory artery produces unilateral deafness

7.8 Insulin-like growth factor-1 (IGF-1):

(a) Increases during pubertal growth spurt
(b) Is a single polypeptide chain
(c) Is produced in pancreas
(d) Is secreted in a pulsatile manner
(e) Is albumin bound in the circulation

7.9 Regarding cystic fibrosis:

(a) It is inherited as autosomal recessive
(b) There is increased risk of bronchial carcinoma in late adulthood
(c) Biliary cirrhosis is a recognised feature
(d) In neonates, intestinal obstruction may be the first presentation
(e) Sweat sodium is decreased

7.10 Hypothalamic nuclei are responsible for:

(a) Control of hunger
(b) Temperature control
(c) Maintaining osmolarity of extracellular fluid
(d) Secretion of thyrotrophin
(e) Control of thyrotrophin secretion

7.11 Adverse effects of NSAIDs include:

(a) Acute renal dysfunction
(b) Renal papillary necrosis
(c) Fluid retention
(d) Hypokalaemia
(e) Nephrotic syndrome

7.12 In a patient with painful joint swelling the following investigations are diagnostic:

(a) C-reactive protein
(b) Antinuclear antibodies
(c) Serum C3 (complement) levels
(d) Microscopic examination of synovial fluid
(e) Factor IX assay

7.13 Complement C3 levels are decreased in:

(a) Systemic lupus erythematoses
(b) Henoch–Schoenlein purpura
(c) Haemolytic uraemic syndrome
(d) Type II membrano-proliferative glomerulonephritis
(e) Focal segmental glomerulosclerosis

7.14 In common variable immunodeficiency (CVID):

(a) Cells are totally absent
(b) Autosomal recessive inheritance may be seen
(c) IgA levels are characteristically normal
(d) T lymphocytes are usually affected
(e) There is increased incidence of autoimmune disorders in families of affected members

7.15 Increased left ventricular end diastolic volume is seen in:

(a) Mitral regurgitation
(b) Congestive cardiomyopathy
(c) Hypertrophic obstructive cardiomyopathy
(d) Aortic stenosis
(e) Pericardial effusion

7.16 Recognised features of constrictive pericarditis are:

(a) Increased fatiguability
(b) Precordial pain
(c) Abdominal distension
(d) Parasternal heave
(e) Pulsatile liver

7.17 FISH is helpful in diagnosing:

(a) Prader-Willi syndrome
(b) Di George syndrome
(c) Klinefelter's syndrome
(d) Turner's syndrome
(e) Angelman syndrome

7.18 In normal neonates:

(a) Extracellular fluid volume exceeds intracellular fluid volume
(b) In a term baby, plasma calcium levels exceed that of the mother
(c) Clamping the umbilical cord after cessation of cord pulsations increases the blood volume by 20%in the baby
(d) There are two arteries and one vein in the umbilical cord
(e) The kidney concentrates urine to an osmolarity that is four times that of plasma

7.19 The following features are more suggestive of biliary atresia rather than neonatal hepatitis in an infant 6 weeks of age:

(a) Hepatomegaly
(b) Prolonged INR (prothrombin time)
(c) Biopsy specimen showed proliferation of bile ductules, periportal fibrosis and bile lakes
(d) HIDA scan reveals delayed uptake and excretion of the contrast material
(e) Ultrasonography reveals absence of gallbladder

7.20 Regarding resuscitation of a three-year old with asystole:

(a) Hypoxia is the commonest cause
(b) It commonly leads to ventricular fibrillation
(c) Intracardiac adrenaline is an absolute indication
(d) IV calcium gluconate is the first line of therapy
(e) The cardiac compressions to respirations ratio is 15:1

7.21 One-year-old child:

(a) Holds a raisin with a finger and thumb
(b) Drinks with a straw
(c) Tells six words with meaning
(d) Can move around holding onto furniture (cruising)
(e) Waves goodbye

7.22 The following are suggestive of abnormal language development:

(a) Not localising sound at 4 months of age
(b) No response to human words at 6 weeks
(c) Not understanding 'no' at 18 months of age
(d) Does not move to music at 2 years of age
(e) Not naming three colours by 4 years of age

7.23 Deafness can develop due to:

(a) Unconjugated hyperbilirubinaemia in the newborn
(b) Pneumococcal meningitis
(c) Alport syndrome
(d) Cleft palate
(e) Gentamicin therapy

7.24 Peak expiratory flow rate:

(a) Is a sensitive parameter to assess improvement to therapy in acute bronchial asthma
(b) Measures small airway resistance
(c) Is more related to height rather than age
(d) Less than 50% of normal is an indication for aminophylline therapy in acute asthma
(e) Is effort independent

7.25 Features differentiating renal tubular acidosis type II from type I include:

(a) Increased anion gap
(b) Nephrocalcinosis
(c) Urinary pH can be lowered < 5.5 in ammonium chloride loading test in type I
(d) Aminoaciduria
(e) Growth failure

7.26 Features of congenital rubella syndrome include:

(a) Intrauterine growth retardation
(b) Hepatomegaly
(c) Thrombocytopenia
(d) Polydactyly
(e) Athetoid cerebral palsy

7.27 *Toxoplasma gondii* infection in humans causes:

(a) Oral ulcers
(b) Cervical lymphadenopathy
(c) Microcephaly
(d) Chorioretinitis
(e) Sacroiliitis

7.28 Epiphyseal changes are seen in:

(a) Non-accidental injury
(b) Rickets
(c) Chronic renal failure
(d) Lead poisoning
(e) Conradi syndrome

7.29 Contributing features to renal osteodystrophy include:

(a) Hypophosphataemia
(b) Hyperparathyroidism
(c) Increased loss of calcium in the kidney
(d) Hypoalbuminaemia
(e) Increased levels of 25-OH cholecalciferol

7.30 X-linked conditions include:

(a) Duchenne muscular dystrophy
(b) Hypophosphataemic rickets
(c) Huntington's chorea
(d) Phenylketonuria
(e) Hunter's disease

Section 8

8.1 The following antibodies are seen in the conditions mentioned:

(a) Anti-endomysial antibodies in coeliac disease
(b) Anti-insulin receptor antibodies in diabetes mellitus
(c) Anti-epidermal antibodies in vitiligo
(d) Anti-acetylcholine receptor antibodies in spinal muscular atrophy
(e) Double-stranded DNA antibodies in SLE

8.2 Recognised features of myotonic dystrophy include:

(a) Phenomenon of anticipation
(b) Muscle pain
(c) Diplopia
(d) Cardiomyopathy
(e) Pseudohypertrophy

8.3 Corneal opacities are seen in:

(a) Marfan's syndrome
(b) Herpes simplex infection
(c) Hurler syndrome
(d) Osteogenesis imperfecta
(e) Ectodermal dysplasia

8.4 Malabsorption may be seen in:

(a) Ischaemia of the gut
(b) Jejunal diverticulosis
(c) Lymphoma of the ileum
(d) Chronic lead poisoning
(e) Giardiasis

8.5 Features of severe folate deficiency include:

(a) Steatorrhoea
(b) Glossitis
(c) Leucoerythroblastic picture
(d) Increased total iron binding capacity
(e) Hypersegmentation of neutrophils

8.6 Spread of hepatitis C occurs by:

(a) Drug abuse
(b) Seafood consumption
(c) Recombinant factor VIII therapy
(d) Faeco-oral spread
(e) Blood transfusion

8.7 A two-year-old child should have been immunised against:

(a) Tetanus
(b) Polio
(c) Measles
(d) Hepatitis A
(e) *Pneumococcus*

8.8 In statistical methodology:

(a) The median and mean are different when the population distribution is skewed
(b) Mode refers to the value that occurs with the highest frequency
(c) The value of 'r' (coefficient of variation) ranges from -1 to $+1$
(d) Incidence is defined as the number of cases seen in the population at any given period of time
(e) The probability that a given result could have been obtained purely by chance is higher when the 'p'-value is 0.01 rather than 0.05

8.9 Increased anion gap is seen in:

(a) Uraemia
(b) Starvation
(c) Renal tubular acidosis
(d) Acetazolamide therapy
(e) Diarrhoea

8.10   In congenital hypertrophic pyloric stenosis:

(a) Conjugated hyperbilirubinaemia may be seen
(b) Hypokalaemia is due to vomiting
(c) Blood pH is high and urinary pH is low
(d) First-born males are commonly affected
(e) Barium swallow is a prerequisite for surgery

8.11   Right to left shunts include:

(a) Fallot's tetralogy
(b) Tricuspid atresia
(c) Eisenmenger complex
(d) Ductus arteriosus in the fetus
(e) ASD as adolescents

8.12   Recognised causes of stroke in children include:

(a) Sickle cell disease
(b) Cystinuria
(c) SLE
(d) Left-to-right shunts
(e) Blunt trauma in mouth

8.13   A psychiatric referral is warranted in a preschool child with the following:

(a) Night terrors
(b) Separation anxiety
(c) Scared of ghosts
(d) Masturbation
(e) Likes to sleep with toys

8.14   Regarding IUGR:

(a) GH deficiency is a recognised complication in later life
(b) Abdominal circumference measured by USG is a diagnostic parameter
(c) Perinatal morbidity is higher in asymmetric IUGR
(d) Nutritional factor is the commonest cause of IUGR in the UK
(e) TSH is decreased

8.15 Benign Rolandic seizures:

(a) Usually occurs at night
(b) Are difficult to control with drugs
(c) Centrotemporal spikes in EEG are a recognised feature
(d) Are more common than petit mal
(e) Start in preschool age

8.16 In febrile convulsions:

(a) Familial predisposition is the same as in idiopathic epilepsy
(b) Carbamazepine achieves good seizure control
(c) *Shigella* dysentery may be a cause
(d) Deafness can occur if seizure is prolonged
(e) Occurs more commonly in girls than boys

8.17 Regarding intussusception in childhood:

(a) Incidence is most common in children over 3 years of age
(b) Barium enema is the investigation of choice
(c) Patient commonly presents with constant abdominal pain
(d) It is associated with Henoch–Schoenlein purpura
(e) Blood in the stools is a must for diagnosis

8.18 Acute laryngotracheobronchitis in children:

(a) Needs to be treated by broad-spectrum antibiotics
(b) Humidified oxygen by tent needs to be administered in infancy
(c) Dexamethasone is known to shorten the duration of illness
(d) Adrenaline by nebuliser is absolutely contraindicated
(e) Viruses are the commonest aetiology

8.19 In scabies:

(a) Itching is due to sensitisation by the mite
(b) Vesicles may be seen in children
(c) The organism is easily demonstrated
(d) Spread can occur through clothes and bedding
(e) The whole family should be treated

8.20   Causes of uveitis include:

(a) Diabetes
(b) Behçet's disease
(c) Ankylosing spondylitis
(d) Rheumatic fever
(e) Inflammatory bowel disease

8.21   Features of severe haemophilia A include:

(a) Retroperitoneal bleed
(b) Chronic arthropathy
(c) Prolonged bleeding time
(d) Increased APTT
(e) Petechial rash

8.22   Gingival hyperplasia is an adverse effect of therapy with:

(a) Phenytoin
(b) Cyclophosphamide
(c) Frusemide
(d) Carbamazepine
(e) Valproate

8.23   Increased fetal haemoglobin is seen in:

(a) Haemoglobin H disease
(b) β-Thalassaemia major
(c) Fanconi's anaemia
(d) Pyruvate kinase deficiency
(e) Hereditary spherocytosis

8.24   Recognised features of anorexia nervosa include:

(a) T-wave inversion on ECG
(b) Hypocholesterolaemia
(c) Peripheral oedema
(d) Sinus bradycardia
(e) Increased plasma cortisol level

8.25 Regarding malaria:

(a) *Plasmodium ovale* has an exoerythrocytic cycle
(b) *Plasmodium malariae* does not occur after 5 years of primary illness
(c) Chloroquine is useful for prophylaxis of falciparum malaria in all areas of the world
(d) Primaquine is used to eradicate falciparum malaria
(e) Parasite load is associated with prognosis

8.26 Renin:

(a) Is secreted mainly in extrarenal tissues
(b) Secretion increases on lying supine
(c) Secretion increases with potassium
(d) Converts angiotensin I into angiotensin II
(e) Secretion regulates osmolality

8.27 Regarding reflex anoxic seizures in children:

(a) ECG-rhythm strip is a must
(b) Asystole may be associated
(c) There is increased risk of epilepsy in adults
(d) Carbamazepine is the drug of choice
(e) Trauma is a well-known precipitating factor

8.28 Regarding idiopathic thrombocytopenic purpura (ITP):

(a) The more severe the disease, the faster is the recovery to therapy
(b) Alloimmunisation occurs due to fetomaternal incompatibility
(c) Splenomegaly is a recognised feature
(d) All children with platelet count less than 50,000 need to be hospitalised
(e) IV immunoglobulin is indicated in all cases

8.29 Indications for an exchange transfusion include:

(a) ABO incompatibility
(b) Acute chest syndrome
(c) Sepsis
(d) Polycythaemia
(e) Sickle nephropathy

8.30 Rare causes of bloody diarrhoea include:

(a) *Campylobacter* infection
(b) *Shigella*
(c) Enterotoxigenic *E. coli*
(d) Crohn's disease
(e) Peutz–Jegher's syndrome

Section 9

9.1 Mitochondrial DNA:

(a) Has its own genome
(b) Is inherited from the father
(c) Can transmit diseases from parents to children
(d) Is present in neurons
(e) Is responsible for some forms of myopathies

9.2 Recognised features in Marfan's syndrome include:

(a) Mutation in fibrillin gene
(b) Sitting height is more than 97th centile
(c) Cognitive impairment
(d) Myopia
(e) Mitral valve prolapse

9.3 Injury to radial nerve involves:

(a) Abductor pollicis brevis is affected
(b) Loss of triceps jerk occurs
(c) Sensory loss on the medial aspect of forearm is seen
(d) First dorsal interosseus is affected
(e) Abduction at the shoulder joint is impaired

9.4 Duchenne muscular dystrophy (DMD):

(a) Affects dystrophin gene
(b) Lens opacities are recognised
(c) Frontal baldness occurs
(d) Is part of the differential diagnosis in a floppy infant
(e) Features usually present before five years of age

9.5   Hereditary angioneurotic oedema (HANE):

(a) Deficiency of Cl esterase occurs
(b) Can present as recurrent abdominal pain
(c) C4 is increased
(d) Androgen agonists are helpful in management
(e) Is transmitted by autosomal recessive inheritance

9.6   Regarding sumatriptan:

(a) It has a good oral bioavailability
(b) Its onset of action is within 15 minutes of subcutaneous administration
(c) Is a 5-HT agonist
(d) Acts on adrenergic and muscarinic receptors
(e) Is used in prophylaxis of migraine

9.7   Regarding immunoglobins:

(a) IgG_2 concentrations increase with age
(b) IgD is useful in mediating the late features of allergic reactions
(c) IgG_2 subclass deficiency is associated with IgA deficiency
(d) IgM is complement-fixing antibody
(e) Type IV hypersensitivity is mediated by IgE

9.8   Common diseases presenting as a rash in infancy are:

(a) Measles
(b) Parvovirus B19 infection
(c) Leukaemia
(d) Lymphoma
(e) Histiocytosis

9.9   Recognised features of brucellosis include:

(a) Osteomyelitis
(b) Liver granuloma
(c) Pericarditis
(d) Splenomegaly
(e) Chronic fatigue

9.10 Water excretion:

(a) Is influenced by the proximal tubule
(b) Is influenced by vasopressin
(c) Depends on erythropoietin
(d) Is influenced by the ascending limb of the loop of Henle
(e) Is influenced by the distal tubule integrity

9.11 Proximal renal tubular functions include:

(a) HCO_3^- secretion
(b) Amino acid absorption
(c) Ammonia production
(d) Urine concentration
(e) Sodium reabsorption

9.12 Growth hormone secretion is raised by:

(a) Sleep
(b) Stress
(c) IGF-1
(d) Somatostatin
(e) Hyperglycaemia

9.13 The following statements are true regarding a screening test:

(a) Sensitivity indicates the proportion of true positives
(b) Specificity indicates the proportion of true negatives
(c) Sensitivity is inversely related to specificity
(d) Prevalence affects predictive value
(e) A good screening test is usually expensive

9.14 Skin lesions characteristically associated with CNS problems:

(a) Dermatitis herpetiformis
(b) Vitiligo
(c) Strawberry angioma on face
(d) Axillary freckling
(e) Periungual fibroma

9.15 Factors triggering renin stimulation:

(a) Hyponatraemia
(b) ACTH
(c) Hypovolaemia
(d) ANP
(e) ADH

9.16 The following are potent vasoconstrictors:

(a) Renin
(b) Angiotensin I
(c) Nitric oxide
(d) PGI_2
(e) ANP

9.17 Long-chain triglyceride absorption requires:

(a) Intraluminal bile salts
(b) PH less than 5
(c) Intraluminal trypsin
(d) Intact duodenum
(e) Mixed micelle formation

9.18 The following statements are true:

(a) EBV causes lymphoma in immunocompromised individuals
(b) Coxsackie virus causes hand, foot and mouth disease
(c) Parvovirus B19 causes haemolytic crisis in sickle cell disease
(d) Human herpes virus 6 is a common cause of rash
(e) Molluscum contagiosum is a viral disease

9.19 The following are recognised in coeliac disease:

(a) Oesophageal carcinoma
(b) Malignant lymphoma
(c) Hyposplenism
(d) Amyloidosis
(e) Vitamin deficiencies

9.20 Increased TSH is seen in a neonate with:

(a) Thyroxine insensitivity
(b) Iodine deficiency
(c) Hyperbilirubinaemia
(d) Thyroid agenesis
(e) Maternal Graves' disease

9.21 Characteristic indices in anaemia of chronic inflammation:

(a) Increased MCV
(b) Decreased ferritin
(c) Decreased transferrin
(d) Normal MCHC
(e) Raised RBC numbers

9.22 Hemolytic anaemia is characterised by:

(a) Increased haptoglobin
(b) Haemosiderinuria
(c) Polychromasia
(d) Megaloblastic bone marrow
(e) Bilirubin present in urine

9.23 In ventricular arrythmia:

(a) PR interval is prolonged
(b) Common in thyrotoxicosis
(c) Synchronised DC shock is the treatment of choice
(d) IV adenosine treatment is effective
(e) QRS duration is normal

9.24 Clinical diagnostic clues in an adolescent female with chronic cough:

(a) Pale stools and diarrhoea
(b) *Aspergillus* precipitin positive
(c) Calcified bronchopulmonary lymph nodes
(d) Whooping cough in the past
(e) Dextrocardia

9.25 Decreased DLCO is seen with:

(a) Increased CO in circulation
(b) Anaemia
(c) Pulmonary fibrosis
(d) Exercise
(e) Emphysema

9.26 The following are true:

(a) Tissue plasminogen activator is derived from endothelium
(b) Heparin acts through antithrombin III
(c) Protein C deficiency is autosomal recessive transmitted
(d) Protein C is vitamin K dependent
(e) Protein S inhibits the action of protein C

9.27 In the most common type of CAH:

(a) Autosomal dominant transmission occurs
(b) 11β-Hydroxylase is deficient
(c) Hypertension is seen
(d) 17-OH progesterone is increased
(e) Increased cortisol levels are seen

9.28 Regarding cisapride:

(a) It is licensed for use in children
(b) Fatal arrythmias have been reported
(c) Concurrent administration with erythromycin is not advised
(d) It commonly causes constipation
(e) Increases gastric emptying time

9.29 Medical treatment of myasthenia gravis includes:

(a) Thymectomy
(b) Physostigmine
(c) Edrophonium
(d) Anticholinergic agents
(e) Steroids

9.30 Diagnosis of nocturnal enuresis can be made in:

(a) A 3-year-old boy with recurrent bedwetting
(b) A 4-year-old who has started bedwetting after attaining complete toilet control at 3½-years of age
(c) A 5-year-old girl who is recently staining her underclothes at school
(d) A 6-year-old recovering from a recent UTI
(e) A 10-year-old girl with recently diagnosed IDDM

Section 10

10.1   The following syndromes are due to chromosomal abnormalities:

(a) Cri-du-chat syndrome
(b) Kearns–Sayre syndrome
(c) Marfan's syndrome
(d) Turner's syndrome
(e) Homocystinuria

10.2   Recognised features in Ehlers–Danlos syndrome include:

(a) Mutation in fibrillin gene
(b) Short stature
(c) Keratoconus
(d) Easy scarring
(e) Mitral valve prolapse

10.3   The following foramina are found in the brain:

(a) Foramen of Monro
(b) Foramen ovale
(c) Foramen of Magendie
(d) Foramen transversalis
(e) Foramen of Luschka

10.4   Common presenting features of myotonic dystrophy are:

(a) Floppy infant
(b) Corneal opacities
(c) Frontal baldness
(d) Macro-orchidism
(e) Microcephaly

10.5 Defects of complement system should be suspected in:

(a) Recurrent folliculitis
(b) Facial swelling following trauma
(c) Recurrent meningococcal infection
(d) *Pneumocystis carinii* pneumonia
(e) Delayed separation of the umbilical cord

10.6 Acetazolamide:

(a) Is used in the management of renal tubular acidosis
(b) Causes hypokalaemia
(c) Is usually given intravenously
(d) Inhibits the action of carbonic anhydrase
(e) Causes metabolic alkalosis

10.7 The following statements about immunoglobulins are false:

(a) IgG is not transferable across the placenta
(b) IgM is usually a pentamer
(c) IgE levels are raised in parasitic infestations
(d) IgD is important in antibody dependent cytotoxicity
(e) IgA deficiency is commoner than agammaglobulinaemia

10.8 Sodium valproate is used in all types of seizures except:

(a) Absences
(b) Infantile spasms
(c) Generalised clonic seizures
(d) Myoclonic type
(e) Status epilepticus

10.9 Respiratory pathogens in the immunosuppressed include:

(a) *Staphylococcus aureus*
(b) *Legionella*
(c) *Pneumocystis carinii*
(d) *Chlamydia*
(e) *Coxiella burnetti*

10.10 Proteins found in muscle fibres include:

(a) Vimentin
(b) Saccharin
(c) Keratin
(d) Desmin
(e) Dystrophin

10.11 The diagnosis of CF can be made by:

(a) A positive family history alone
(b) Raised sweat $Na^+ > 40\,mmol/l$
(c) Positive genetic study
(d) Raised serum levels of trypsinogen
(e) Stool lipase

10.12 Presenting features of gastro-oesophageal reflux in infants include:

(a) Vomiting
(b) Apnoeas
(c) Tachypnoea
(d) Poor feeding
(e) Persistent crying

10.13 The following statements are true regarding a normal distribution curve:

(a) The median is the same as the mean
(b) $2 \times SD$ represents 98% of the sample values
(c) Parametric tests are used in statistical analysis
(d) It is not possible to calculate the mode
(e) All variables can be represented in this fashion

10.14 Differential diagnosis of seborrhoeic dermatitis in infancy includes:

(a) Eczema
(b) Psoriasis
(c) Icthyosis
(d) Candidiasis
(e) Contact dermatitis

10.15 Growth hormone secretion is influenced by:

(a) Sleep
(b) GHRH (growth hormone releasing hormone)
(c) IGF-2
(d) Somatostatin
(e) Hypoglycaemia

10.16 Common vasculitides in childhood include:

(a) Polyarteritis nodosa
(b) Henoch–Schoenlein purpura
(c) SLE
(d) Kawasaki disease
(e) Churg–Strauss syndrome

10.17 Prolonged TPN can cause all except:

(a) Abnormal liver functions
(b) Zinc deficiency
(c) Hypoglycaemia
(d) Rickets of prematurity
(e) Hyponatraemia

10.18 The following statements are true:

(a) *Aspergillus* can cause systemic disease in immunocompromised hosts
(b) Mucormycosis is common in diabetic children
(c) *Candida* infection is recognised by the presence of spores on microscopy
(d) *Microsporum canis* causes scalp infections
(e) Molluscum contagiosum is a fungal disease

10.19 Type I diabetes is a feature of:

(a) DIDMOAD syndrome
(b) Polyglandular autoimmune disease type I
(c) Polyglandular autoimmune disease type II
(d) Schmidt syndrome
(e) Haemochromatosis

10.20 Recognised actions of theophylline in apnoea of prematurity include:

(a) On respiratory centre
(b) Promoting diaphragmatic movement
(c) On intercostal muscles
(d) Stimulating vagal activity
(e) Antagonism to adenosine

10.21 Causes of aplastic anaemia include:

(a) Fanconi syndrome
(b) Hepatitis B infection
(c) Down's syndrome
(d) Carbamazepine
(e) EBV infection

10.22 The following tumours are very radiosensitive:

(a) Medulloblastoma
(b) Acute lymphoblastic leukemia
(c) Ewing sarcoma
(d) Wilm's tumour
(e) Osteosarcoma

10.23 Normal findings in the ECG of an 8-month-old girl:

(a) T-wave inversion in V1 and V2
(b) PR interval 0.25 s
(c) Axis +126°
(d) QT interval 0.34 s
(e) P-wave 2 mV

10.24 Clinical diagnostic clues in an adolescent female with delayed puberty include:

(a) Short stature
(b) Weight loss and abdominal pain
(c) Multiple large café-au-lait spots
(d) Lanugo hair and low temperature
(e) Family history of delayed puberty

10.25 Reduced FEF$_{25-75}$ is an indicator of:

(a) Asthma
(b) Cystic fibrosis
(c) Kyphoscoliosis
(d) Bronchiectasis
(e) Croup

10.26 The following are true statements:

(a) Unexplained vaginal discharge in a 3-year-old might be a sign of sexual abuse
(b) Spiral fracture of femur is always non-accidental
(c) Retinal bleeding in a 3-month-old unconscious baby is a sign of 'shaken baby' syndrome
(d) Bruises on the elbows and knees in a 4-year-old are suggestive of physical abuse
(e) Masturbation in a 5-year-old girl is a sign of sexual abuse

10.27 In autism:

(a) Social interaction is normal
(b) Dopamine levels are reduced
(c) Genetic factors may play a role in aetiology
(d) Methylphenidate is used with benefit
(e) Tantrums are common

10.28 Frequent complications of *Mycoplasma* infection include:

(a) Thrombocytopenia
(b) Haemolytic anaemia
(c) Cardiac conduction defects
(d) Pleural effusion
(e) Guillain–Barré syndrome

10.29 Elevated levels of CPK are seen in:

(a) Duchenne muscular dystrophy
(b) Dermatomyositis
(c) Spinal muscular atrophy
(d) Malignant hyperthermia
(e) Neonates

10.30 The following enzymes and inhibitors are matched correctly:

(a) Xanthine oxidase–allopurinol
(b) Enolase–fluoride
(c) Cholinesterase–physostigmine
(d) Ceruloplasmin–penicillamine
(e) Cytochrome P450–phenobarbitone

Answers

Section 1

1.1 (a)
Normal maintenance requirements for the first 10 kg is 100ml for each kilogram, an additional 50 ml/kg for each of the next 10 kg, then 20ml/kg for each extra kilogram. Normal sodium needs are 2–3 mmol/kg/day. A fluid deficit of 50 ml/kg leads to a weight loss of 5%, 100ml/kg 10% and so on. In children, hypotension is a late sign indicative of cardiovascular collapse and severe (15%) dehydration. A child with constant vomiting with pyloric stenosis loses Na, K and Cl from the gastric fluid in addition to H^+ and so, ends up with an alkalosis, with decreased K and Cl.

1.2 (b), (c)
Muscle fasciculations are a sign of damage to the lower motor neurons, i.e. the anterior horn cells. A posterior cord transection would involve the spinothalamic tracts (which carry pain and temperature sensation) and the fibres carrying proprioceptive and fine touch sensations. This would spare the corticospinal tracts. Athetoid movements are involuntary movements produced by the involvement of the basal ganglia. Athetoid cerebral palsy is seen in children with kernicterus, which affects the basal ganglia.

1.3 (a), (b), (c)
Reye syndrome is an anicteric hepatitis and encephalopathy, with acute liver failure. It commonly follows varicella infection/aspirin ingestion, and presents with hypoglycaemia, elevated ammonia levels, and cerebral oedema. Citrullinaemia is a urea cycle defect, methylmalonic acidaemia is an organic acid disorder, and isovaleric acidaemia is an aminoaciduria. Aminoacidurias do not as a general rule present with hyperammonaemia, organic acidaemias may.

1.4 (a), (d), (e)
MGN presents rarely in children (common in the second decade of life). When it does, it presents as nephrotic syndrome, with non-selective proteinuria. The immune complexes are composed of IgG and C3 and are deposited on the epithelial side of the membrane. Serum C3 levels are normal as is the blood pressure. It carries a worse prognosis in children

with nephrotic syndrome. The disease may also occur secondary to SLE, Hepatitis B virus infection and gold or penicillamine therapy.

1.5 (b)
Jaundice in a 12-hour-old neonate is uncommon, and the common causes of this are Rhesus/ABO isoimmunisation. G6PD deficiency leads to prolonged jaundice/high bilirubin levels after the first 24 hours. Criggler Najjar syndrome is of 2 types. Type I is mild; type II is autosomal recessively inherited and is the severe form of the disease, with complete absence of UDP glucuronyl transferase, the enzyme responsible for conjugating the lipid-soluble bilirubin to make it water soluble and able to be excreted in the urine and stool. It may result in early severe jaundice, but is very rare. Choledochal cyst causes direct hyperbilirubinaemia later in the newborn period.

1.6 (b), (d)
UTIs are commoner in uncircumcised male infants than girls, but after that age group, there is no difference in the incidence of UTIs between girls and boys. VUR is usually a cause of UTI rather than a result. *E. coli* is the commonest organism isolated from UTIs. Risk factors include constipation, neurological problems involving the bladder and bowel (spina bifida, operated sacro-coocygeal teratoma, etc). Long-term trimethoprim is usually used to prevent further infections until investigations prove no underlying cause for the UTI in children less than 5 years of age.

1.7 (c), (d), (e)
Acute liver failure is characterised by Reye syndrome, acute fulminant hepatitis from drugs/viruses. Wilson's disease is rare, and usually presents with liver failure or hepatitis, associated with development of behavioural problems/psychiatric disturbances/other neurological symptoms later on in childhood. Extrahepatic biliary atresia is a remediable cause of liver failure – a Kasai operation is performed early in the course of the disease.

1.8 (c), (e)
Indications for an exchange transfusion reaction in a child with sickle cell disease may include an acute CNS event (stroke), priapism, acute chest syndrome and a vaso-occlusive crisis (VOC) refractory to initial management – analgesia, fluids, correction of acidosis and oxygen. Splenic sequestration is

managed with a packed red cell transfusion, as is an aplastic crisis. Dactylitis is a form of VOC. Chronic exchange transfusional programmes to keep HbS < 30% may be necessary after an acute CNS event or in cardiomyopathy.

1.9 (a), (b), (c), (d), (e)
Chronic exposure of the fetus to high blood glucose from the mother induces insulin production, and the resultant hyperinsulinism causes initial hypoglycaemia. Hypocalcaemia is common, and so is polycythaemia leading to jaundice.

1.10 (d), (e)
SLE is commoner in the second decade of life, although younger children may be affected. The disease is characterised by production of antibodies to many nuclear, serum and cytoplasmic proteins. Antibodies to double-stranded DNA are the most specific. This is often coincident with a low C3 and C4 and indicates renal disease. Multi-system involvement shows up as varied symptoms and signs including facial 'butterfly' rash, purpura, telangiectasia, Raynaud's phenomenon, alopecia, photosensitivity, anaemia, thrombocytopenia and lymphopenia, renal involvement and joint and serous membrane involvement (pericardial effusion, pleural effusion and arthritis). Renal disease prognosis is variable and reaches a 90% 10 year survival with treatment.

1.11 (a), (d), (e)
Rett syndrome is a neurodegenerative disorder occurring only in females, with suspected X-linked dominant inheritance. Development is normal until a year of age, after which acquired microcephaly occurs with delay in motor and language milestones. Characteristic features to remember are sighing respirations with intermittent apnoeas, repetitive hand movements, autistic behaviour, and generalised seizures.

1.12 (a), (b), (c), (e)

1.13 (a), (b), (d), (e)
Clubbing is seen as a response to systemic hypoxaemia in many conditions. Pulmonary causes include suppurative conditions like abscess and bronchiectasis, carcinoma and interstitial fibrosis. Cardiac causes include cyanotic heart disease with a right to left shunting and infective endocarditis. Gastrointestinal causes include inflammatory bowel disease

like Crohn's and ulcerative colitis.

1.14 (c), (e)

Guillain–Barré syndrome (GBS) is an immune mediated polyneuropathy that follows a viral trigger in most cases. Motor involvement is common. There are rarely any definite sensory changes in GBS although there may be paraesthesia in the initial stages of the illness. Muscle wasting is not seen. CSF may be normal in the initial stages and then present with high protein content and normal cell counts. External ophthalmoplegia is found as an uncommon variant.

1.15   (b), (c)

Recurrent abdominal pain is common in children in older age groups and in adolescence. The pain is non-specific and symptoms have lasted for more than 3 months at presentation. Organic causes include *Helicobacter pylori* infection, abdominal migraine and constipation. Although all the causes listed can cause recurrent abdominal pain, the common ones are constipation and functional causes. Prognosis is fairly good, although many children develop irritable bowel syndrome as adults.

1.16   (a), (c)

Tricky wording! Note the word *primary* – so choice (d) is out. A tachypnoeic baby has a lung problem accounting for hypoxia, and a TGA (transposition of great arteries) can present as choice (e). A certain diagnosis can be made only in (a) and (c).

1.17   (b)

Less than 10% of the cases of juvenile chronic arthritis (JCA) have positive RF. A more useful antibody to test for is the anti-nuclear factor (ANF), which is seen in most children with pauci-articular JCA. Cervical spine involvement is as common as 50% of cases. The first line drugs are NSAIDs, then low-dose methotrexate is considered. There is no reliable indicator for the development of chronic uveitis and therefore regular slit lamp examinations are indicated in pauci-articular arthritis to detect early uveitis.

1.18   (b), (e)

1.19   (c)

Penicillins and cephalosporins interfere with cell wall synthesis.

Ciprofloxacin inhibits DNA gyrase and sulpha drugs inhibit folate synthesis in bacteria. Macrolides (erythro-, azithro- and clarithromycin) aminoglycosides and chloramphenicol inhibit translation.

1.20 (d)
There is pulmonary oligaemia in tetralogy of Fallot (due to pulmonary stenosis) and in Eisenmenger's syndrome (due to high pulmonary vascular resistance). Coarctation of the aorta presents with rib notching due to collaterals if left undetected after the neonatal period. There is associated hypertension. *Pneumocystis carinii* infection causes pneumonia.

1.21 (a), (b), (e)
Haemophilia is a deficiency in factor VIII or IX, which are part of the coagulation cascade in the intrinsic pathway. They present with clotting problems and deep bruising rather than petechial spots or gum bleeding which is commoner in platelet defects or diseases typified by poor vascular support (eg Ehlers-Danlos syndrome). Factor VIII does not cross the placenta – neonatal bleeding is therefore possible.

1.22 (a), (b)

1.23 (a), (c), (d), (e)
Isosexual indicates that the secondary sexual characters are for the same sex. McCune–Albright syndrome (polyostotic fibrous dysplasia) is caused by an activating missense mutation in the G protein that stimulates cAMP formation. This disease constitutes hyperpigmented macules, precocious puberty and thinning and fracture of bones. CAH on the other hand causes virilisation in a female. Hypothalamic hamartomas may cause increased secretion of GnRH and contribute to early puberty. However, constitutional cause is the commonest in girls.

1.24 (b), (c), (d)
Dandy–Walker malformation consists of a cystic expansion of the 4th ventricle and causes hydrocephalus. Soto syndrome or cerebral gigantism presents with rapid growth, and infants are usually > 97th centile for length and weight by a year of age and continue to grow rapidly. Mental retardation is common. Rett syndrome is an example of acquired microcephaly and is seen in girls.

1.25   (b), (d), (e)
Trisomy 21 presents with low AFP.

1.26   (a), (b), (c), (e)
Distal/type I renal tubular acidosis (DRTA) is a defect in the distal tubule in acidification of urine. Hypokalaemia is a result of the imbalance in the H^+, K^+, Na^+ pump and impaired hydrogen ion transport. Since this is the main area for acidification, the urine pH is never < 5.5. Secondary causes of DRTA are sickle cell nephropathy, EDS (Ehlers-Danlos syndrome) and lupus nephritis.

1.27   (a), (b), (c), (d), (e)

1.28   (c), (d), (e)
Emergency management of a 4-year-old in coma involves attention to ABC, and a blood sugar. The first two choices are not needed in this situation. The other investigations are only helpful in making a diagnosis.

1.29   (a), (c), (e)
The effects of raised K^+ are on the cardiovascular and the neuromuscular system. It is made worse by acidosis, and is treated if the serum K^+ > 7 or if symptomatic. Typical ECG changes include tall peaked T-waves. First line treatment includes calcium gluconate (to reverse the cardiovascular effects), insulin with dextrose, intravenous salbutamol and the use of resonium–ion exchange resin.

1.30   (b), (c)
Selenium is a trace element, which is now commonly added to TPN, although it was common to find deficiency states in the past. Deficiency causes a form of cardiomyopathy called Keshan disease. Abnormal liver functions and cholestasis are common problems with long-term administration of TPN. Although the exact mechanisms are unknown, intralipid and high concentrations of amino acids are implicated. Osteopenia results from inadequate phosphate, unless supplemented. Hyperglycaemia is more a short-term problem.

Section 2

2.1 (d), (e)

Short-acting insulin acts by 1–4 hours and wanes by 6 hours. Bedtime reading is influenced by the short-acting component of the evening dose, and levels over 7 indicate that it is unlikely to have a hypoglycaemic episode in the night. Lipodystrophy from use of the same site for injection is a cause of poor absorption and consequently increased needs of insulin. HbA1c levels reflect the glycaemic control in the past 2–3 months. Levels are < 7% in normal individuals. In diabetics, > 12% represents poor control, and < 9% adequate control.

2.2 (b), (d)

Immediate referral is indicated for a weight/height < 0.4 centile. Calculation of the midparental height (MPH) is useful to predict the height potential of the child and compare it to existing value. MPH in a boy is Mum + Dad ÷ 2 + 7 cm, and in a girl M + D ÷ 2 – 8.5 cm. The target centile range is obtained by plotting the MPH on the chart and then marking centile ranges 10 cm above and below. An adult predicted height below or above target centile range is abnormal and needs referral. Separate charts exist for children with Turner's and Down's syndromes and in those with achondroplasia.

2.3 (a)

Establishing the diagnosis of coeliac disease is possible only with jejunal biopsy/positive IgA anti-endomysial antibodies. The rest of the tests suggest either malabsorption (72-hour faecal fat) or are non-specific (anti-gliadin antibodies). False-negative results from an antibody screen to endomysial antibodies will result from IgA deficiency, so make sure to check immunoglobulin levels if in doubt.

2.4 (d)

The criteria to diagnose Kawasaki disease include fever > 39°C for > 5 days, non-purulent conjunctivitis, > 2 cm cervical adenopathy bilaterally, mucous membrane involvement in the form of strawberry tongue/lip cracking, skin rash and redness, swelling and peeling of the fingers/toes.

Late changes include the skin peeling, changes in platelet count (thrombocytosis) and development of coronary (sometimes other medium-sized arteries) aneurysms.

2.5   (d)
Generalised absences are typical/atypical, the former being more common. They are usually seen over the age of 4, and occur more frequently in girls. CT scans show abnormalities in < 10% cases. A typical EEG with 3/s spike and wave is characteristic, and the diagnosis is difficult to make in its absence. Hypsarrhythmia is the typical EEG pattern seen in infantile spasms.

2.6   (a), (b), (c)
Werdnig–Hoffman disease is spinal muscular dystrophy type I and involves the anterior horn cells. Guillain–Barré syndrome is an immune poly-radiculopathy and involves motor fibres in the nerve roots. Tertiary syphilis on the other hand causes tabes dorsalis, which is typified by a sensory tract involvement in the fibres carrying fine touch and proprioception. Charcot–Marie–Tooth disease is a hereditary neuropathy, which involves motor and sensory fibres in the peripheral nerve.

2.7   (a), (b)
Although the typical findings in tuberous sclerosis (autosomal dominant inheritance) are ash leaf macules, café-au-lait spots are also seen. Other features of tuberous sclerosis are shagreen patches, periungual fibromas, adenoma sebaceum and phakomas. Neurofibromatosis type I is associated with café-au-lait spots, and these usually have an irregular border (coast of Maine appearance vs. the coast of California appearance in McCune–Albright syndrome). The latter condition is a cause of precocious puberty in girls, but is uncommon. Most girls with precocious puberty have a constitutional cause.

2.8   (c), (e)
Polycythaemia is an uncommon cause of jaundice on the whole, although it is common after physiological jaundice is excluded from the causes. A central venous haematocrit > 65% is significant, and needs a partial exchange transfusion if symptoms such as apnoeas, jitteriness, poor feeding, and seizures coexist. There is hardly any consensus on the long-term benefits of a partial exchange transfusion and some studies have

reported better neurological outcome after the procedure. On the whole, however, only proven short-term benefits of reducing cardiovascular, cerebral and splanchnic haemodynamic effects exist. No long-term benefits are clear.

2.9   (a), (d)
HSV type I causes oral infection, whereas type II causes genital infection. Lichen planus is a skin condition, which is associated with white net like lesions in the oral cavity. Dermatitis herpetiformis is a condition presenting with symmetric, grouped, intensely pruritic papules and vesicles in the buttocks, elbows and knees, with sparing of mucous membranes. Association with gluten-sensitive enteropathy is seen in 75–90% and IgA and C3 deposits are seen in the basement membrane. Most effective treatment is with dapsone.

2.10   (b), (c)
Emergency is the key word here, and oxygen is indicated for the bronchospasm that accompanies an anaphylactic reaction. H_2 receptors are found in the gastric mucosa and examples of blockers are ranitidine/famotidine. Anti-histamines of choice here are H_1 blockers (chlorpheniramine or Piriton). Anaphylaxis is a type I hypersensitivity reaction mediated by mast cells and release of histamine.

2.11   (a), (b), (e)
21-Hydroxylase deficiency is the commonest form of CAH, and presents in two-thirds of cases as the classical salt-losing type, with virilisation due to the excess steroids produced proximal to the defect. Hypertension is a sign found in 11-hydroxylase deficiency, due to the excess deoxycortisol produced prior to the defect. Long-standing VUR leads to scarring of the kidneys and chronic glomerulonephritis and renal failure from reflux nephropathy. Patients with Turner's syndrome may be hypertensive from the coarctation that commonly complicates their condition or as part of the disease in adolescence.

2.12   (b), (d)
Croup is a descriptive term rather than a disease. The commonest cause of croup is viral (parainfluenza). Nebulised budesonide is used now widely for acute relief in croup and reduction of hospital admissions. There is good evidence now that oral and nebulised dexamethasone is as effective

as nebulised budesonide and is much cheaper. Adrenaline is reserved for acute severe airway obstruction, because it usually causes a rebound oedema and worsening symptoms. It is usually reserved for the short duration of time that precedes the decision to intubate and ventilate the child.

2.13   (c)

Paediatric HIV is more than a downsized version of adult HIV infection. Lymphocytic interstitial pneumonitis (LIP), growth and developmental delay, HIV encephalopathy and the rarity of Kaposi sarcoma are some of the differences. In an infant suspected to have HIV, prophylaxis against *Pneumocystis carinii* infection is started as soon as possible and continued until diagnosis is confirmed/refuted. Antenatal screening of mothers is now offered in the UK. This is supported by trials that have shown reduced transplacental transmission of HIV infection by treating the mothers in the second and third trimester (as well as the baby after birth for 6–8 weeks) with anti-retroviral drugs like zidovudine (AZT) and didanosine.

2.14   (b)

Sensitivity is the ability to pick up true positives, and specificity is the ability to minimise false positives. The positive predictive value (PPV) of a test is dependent on the incidence of a particular disease being screened in that population and as such varies even with the same screening test in different populations. Values of greater than 90% specificity are necessary to justify the use of a screening test in common practice. A good screening test is cheap, easy, reproducible, repeatable, screens for a disease for which there is a cure/disease modifying therapy, and one whose disease criteria are well established.

2.15   (b), (c), (e)

Upper airway ends at the level of the cords, and therefore (a) and (d) are not true.

2.16   (a), (b), (c), (d), (e)

2.17   (a), (d)

Sophisticated tests for the hearing screen include the auditory brainstem responses/evoked potentials. These are not used in the community routinely. In the community, distraction test is used routinely around the age of 9 months. It involves two people, one standing in front of the child to distract the child and another behind the child to use an object emitting soft sounds. While the child is thus distracted, the person at the back produces a sound from a 45° angle to one side. The child responds by turning. This is repeated on the other side.

2.18   (a), (c)
Choice (a) demonstrates the dissociation of language and fine motor milestones. Bottom-shufflers are normal variants and they usually show some gross motor delay initially before they catch up.

2.19   (a), (c), (e)
The first sign of puberty in a boy is the enlargement of testicular volume. Prepubertal volume is ~4 ml, and adult volumes ~12 ml. This is tested by using an orchidometer with varying sized beads to indicate the volume. The definition of delayed puberty in boys is lack of pubertal changes by 17 years, and in girls, 15 years. Precocious puberty in boys can result from CAH.

2.20   (a), (b), (e)
The complement cascade is an immunological defence mechanism separate from humoral and cellular immunity, although it works in conjunction with them. It occurs in two pathways – classical and alternate. The final end product is the C5-9 complex, which causes cell lysis. Bacterial endotoxins activate both arms of the pathway. Hereditary angioneurotic oedema is caused by the deficiency of C1 esterase inhibitor, and is an autosomal dominant transmitted disease.

2.21   (a), (b), (d)

2.22   (a), (c)
The routine testing of a child with a UTI < 1-year old (some say < 2-years old) includes an ultrasound scan, DMSA and an MCUG (micturating cystourethrogram). Under 5, children can be managed with a DMSA scan and a renal ultrasound, and a cystogram (indirect/direct) done if there is evidence of scarring. Over 5, there is little possible benefit other than from a renal ultrasound. Prophylaxis is usually reserved for the under 5-year-old child with possible reflux and risk of recurrent infection in the kidneys.

2.23   (a), (b), (e)
(c) and (d) actually inhibit the hepatic cytochrome P 450 system.

2.24   (a)
Kallman syndrome comprises anosmia, hypogonadotropic hypogonadism (HH) and obesity. Testicular atrophy leads to hypergonadotropism. LHRH testing is rarely able to separate HH from constitutional delay. Buserelin is a GnRH agonist, and is not very commonly used in the treatment.

2.25   (c), (d)
Prader Willi syndrome (PWS) is caused by the paternal deletion of a part of chromosome 15, or a uniparental disomy of maternal chromosome 15. This is the exact opposite of Angelman syndrome. (Prader for p = paternal!). This phenomenon of phenotype being influenced by the origin of the chromosome is called genomic imprinting. Other examples include Beckwith–Weidemann syndrome. Infants with PWS are hypotonic, poor feeders and need nasogastric feeding. In childhood, they develop behavioural problems, start overeating, become obese and demonstrate self-picking behaviour. Developmental delay is common. They have a characteristic facies with almond-shaped eyes.

2.26   (a), (b), (c)
Classical autism presents usually before the age of 30 months, with poor social milestones, poor eye contact, characteristic routines and getting extremely upset with changes in routine, repetitive behaviour and poor speech. Prognosis is guarded, with most needing to go into care in adult life.

2.27   (a), (b), (d)
Petit mal has a typical 3 Hz spike and wave activity all over, infantile spasms have chaotic irregular hypsarrhythmic pattern, and herpes encephalitis shows temporal lobe spikes.

2.28   (a), (b), (c)
Fetal ultrasound diagnosis of renal tract anomalies has reached sophisticated levels and the natural history of such abnormalities is only now being elucidated. Causes for a dilated renal collecting system in the foetus include foetal vesico-ureteric reflux, pelvi-ureteric junction obstruction and even a normal variant. Definitions of a dilated renal pelvis include AP

diameter > 5 mm at 20 weeks and > 7 mm at 32 weeks (controversy exists regarding this). A multicystic dysplastic kidney is one with virtually poor function and dilated collecting systems in the form of cysts.

2.29   (b), (c)

Adrenal medulla cells are of neural crest origin. Langerhans cells are skin phagocytes.

2.30   (b), (c), (d)

Section 3

3.1 (a), (c), (e)

Childhood asthma is different from adult asthma in many ways: cough may be the only symptom, especially nocturnal; response to β_2-agonists is poor in infancy (there is anecdotal evidence that ipratropium bromide is better in this age group); and there is a strong association with exercise and activity. Most exacerbations of asthma in childhood are a result of viral URTIs (upper respiratory tract infections); however, allergy to house dust mite and animal fur is an important precipitant. Smoking exacerbates the asthmatic symptoms.

3.2 (b), (d), (e)

Oral rehydration therapy has revolutionised the management of acute diarrhoea. This is based on the fact that sodium and water absorption in the small gut is facilitated by the presence of glucose (a common active transport carrier mechanism) – oral rehydration solutions consist of various ratios of sodium, glucose, and other salts. Breast-feeding should be continued in the face of acute diarrhoea, and IV fluids are necessary only in severe dehydration. Anti-diarrhoeal drugs are to be avoided as they increase the risk of invasive disease. *Salmonella* septicaemia following gastroenteritis is common in neonates, HIV infected children (is a CDC (Communicable Diseases Center, Atlanta, GA, USA) AIDS disease-defining criterion), inflammatory bowel disease and in sickle cell disease.

3.3 (a), (b), (c)

Congenital syphilis presents with symptoms in two phases – early (<2 years) and late. The neonate may be asymptomatic at birth and then present within weeks with hepatosplenomegaly, petechiae, elevated liver enzymes, Coomb's negative haemolytic anaemia, typical osteochondritis and periostitis, skin manifestations like bullae and desquamating macular rash, failure to thrive and rarely nephritic syndrome. Luckily, with increased antenatal care and testing, this is a rarity in developed countries.

3.4 (a), (b), (c), (e)

3.5 (a), (b), (c), (d), (e)

Torsion of the testis is an emergency in infancy – the viability of the testis is greatly influenced by the extent of delay in correcting the torsion. Causes of orchitis include mumps, Coxsackie infection, and in some parts of the world tuberculosis. Beware of a strangulated hernia! A haematocele from a difficult breech delivery would present with a tender, swollen, red scrotum.

3.6 (a), (c), (d)

Term babies are able to fixate light and follow objects horizontally well, by 6 weeks they are able to follow in a circle.

3.7 (b), (c), (e)

Retinoblastoma is the most important cause of leucocoria (white reflex), not leucorrhoea! This leads to heterochromia iridis (difference in pupillary colours). 30% have bilateral disease and an autosomally dominantly inherited predisposition, 20% of the unilateral disease have genetic predisposition. The gene is localised to the long arm of chromosome 13. Standard therapy for unilateral disease is enucleation, and bilateral disease is radiotherapy/cryotherapy.

3.8 (b)

Salt losers presenting in the newborn period with crisis are more likely to be female. The commonest cause of ambiguous genitalia at birth is CAH, of which 95% are deficient in 21-hydroxylase. Less common enzyme defects involve 11β-hydroxylase and 3β-hydroxysteroid dehydrogenase. About two-thirds of those deficient in 21-hydroxylase are salt losers, and present with an Addisonian crisis.

3.9 (b), (d)

Infantile eczema presents usually around the age of 2–3 months. The usual areas to be affected are the cheeks and then the face, wrists, neck and extensor surfaces. Pruritus is marked. The onset coincides with introduction of certain food products like cow's milk, soya, eggs or fish. Overall, a third of patients exhibit food-related hypersensitivity to the major allergens. Resolution of symptoms is common after the age of 5. A positive family history of atopy, elevated serum IgE and the presence of eosinophilia support the diagnosis. Seborrhoeic dermatitis is a common differential diagnosis and may co-exist.

3.10   (d), (e)
Syndromes with hypogonadism and obesity are rare and include Prader-Willi syndrome and Kallman syndrome. Obesity in childhood is increasing and the risk of its persisting into adult life is high (nearly 70% for obese children at the age of 10–13 years). Pathological consequences include low fitness levels, increased blood pressure, low HDL and high total cholesterol, polycystic ovarian disease and adverse social and psychological effects. Relatively tall stature is common in these children.

3.11   (c), (d)

3.12   (a), (c), (e)
Acute bronchiolitis is a lower respiratory infection caused most commonly by respiratory syncitial virus in epidemic fashion most winters. Other viruses like adenovirus, parainfluenza viruses and influenza virus cause infection and a similar clinical picture. It presents most commonly in infancy, infections in later childhood presenting as upper respiratory infection. Respiratory distress is accompanied by fine crackles in the lung bases. Treatment of most uncomplicated infants is with supportive measures like oxygen and nasogastric feeds. At-risk infants, such as those with heart disease or chronic lung disease, may need further treatment in the form of ribavirin used in some units. A recently introduced monoclonal antibody given monthly as prophylaxis (palivizumab) has been shown to reduce hospitalisations by 55%.

3.13   (d)

3.14   (b), (c)
Metabolic alkalosis with hypokalaemia is seen in pyloric stenosis because of the loss of stomach acid with K^+ and HCl, and cystic fibrosis as in pseudo-Bartter syndrome. Bartter syndrome is a form of renal potassium wasting with elevated renin and aldosterone; the K^+ is usually < 2.5 mmol/l. Renal failure and urinary diversion procedures cause metabolic acidosis.

3.15 (a), (c)

Childhood schizophrenia is rare (even in adolescence, incidence is < 3 per 10,000). Delusions, hallucinations, catatonia and thought insertion and withdrawal are common. School performance deteriorates slowly.

3.16 (a), (b), (d)

Spinal muscular atrophy is classified into three forms: infantile, late infantile and juvenile. The specific gene defect (autosomal recessive inheritance) is localised to chromosome 5, which in the defective state fails to suppress the normal pre-programmed neuronal cell death at birth. The characteristic features are fasciculations seen best in the resting tongue, fibrillation potentials in EMG and denervation pattern on a muscle biopsy.

3.17 (a), (b), (d)

3.18 (b), (e)

3.19 (a) (d), (e)

Bronchiolitis is a disease of infancy and early childhood caused by RSV in most epidemics. Many infants wheeze after this first episode, with viral URTIs. It is an infection of terminal bronchioles and therefore causes air trapping and wheeze. No drug therapy has shown to be of significant benefit, although bronchodilators may work in some cases. Ribavirin is restricted to high-risk groups like ex-premature infants, infants with heart disease, infants with significant respiratory problems like broncho-pulmonary dysplasia, etc. Newer treatments to prevent infection in high-risk groups include monoclonal antibodies (palivizumab), which are still being tested in routine clinical practice.

3.20 (b), (e)

3.21 (b), (c)

3.22 (c)

Salbutamol causes hypokalaemia, and is used in acute treatment of hyperkalaemia. Digoxin by itself does not cause any hypokalaemia, although the effects of the drug on the heart are exacerbated in the presence of low serum potassium. ACE inhibitors cause hyperkalaemia.

3.23   (a), (b), (c), (d), (e)

3.24   (b), (c), (d), (e)
Herpes encephalitis has a very poor prognosis in its full-blown form. Death is common and in survivors, severe neurological sequelae are common. Temporal lobes are selectively affected and an EEG would reveal bitemporal spikes. MRI or CT scans would show density in bilateral temporal lobes. Post-infectous encephalitis in varicella infection is cerebellar and presents with ataxia, nystagmus and poor co-ordination. It is self-correcting and has a good prognosis.

3.25   (a), (b), (c), (d)
Falciparum malaria is complicated by hypoglycaemia, CNS involvement, renal failure from either haemolysis or directly, and gastrointestinal damage. Leptospira infection causes Weil's disease, which primarily affects the liver, kidneys and blood.

3.26   (a), (b), (d), (e)
In intravascular haemolysis, haemoglobinuria occurs as a result of breakdown of red cells in the intravascular space. This presents with dark-coloured urine, which tests positive on dipstix for blood, but reveals no red cells on microscopy.

3.27   (a), (c), (d)

3.28   (c)
Achondroplasia is an autosomal dominant inherited condition, although many are a result of new mutations. Infertility is not a feature. The limbs are shortened in disproportion to the spine in this skeletal dysplasia.

3.29   (a), (e)

3.30   (b)

Section 4

4.1 (b), (c), (e)
Prematurity is the most important risk factor for NEC, although high-risk neonates have a higher chance of developing NEC – umbilical artery catheters, asphyxia, sepsis, rapid feeding patterns and high osmolality feeds have all been implicated. Hirschsprung's disease predisposes to enterocolitis in the dilated bowel proximal to the aganglionic part. The risk of enterocolitis in Hirschsprung's disease is not reduced even after surgery and only reduces with increasing age, possibly related to an evolving mucous barrier with age.

4.2 (a), (c), (e)
Down's syndrome is Trisomy 21, caused in most cases by non-separation of the chromosomes at meiosis. This is the commonest chromosomal disorder in the general population with an incidence of 1 in 800 live births. In 4% of cases, reciprocal translocations are seen to cause the disease and therefore there is a recurrence risk. Hypotonia, brachycephaly, neck folds, wide space between first and second toes, simian crease, clinodactyly, and the typical facies with mongoloid slant and epicanthic folds support the diagnosis. There is an increased risk of cataracts, leukaemias and myelodysplasia with Trisomy 21.

4.3 (a), (d)
Metabolism of the rest of the drugs is by the liver primarily. Metalozone is a strong diuretic.

4.4 (b), (c)
NSAIDs are contraindicated in children with asthma because they may cause further bronchoconstriction.

4.5 (c)
Distal renal tubular acidosis (RTA) or type I RTA presents as a failure to acidify urine below pH 5.5 even on loading with ammonium chloride owing to a defect in H^+ ion secretion in the distal tubule. It can occur in adults and children. In infants, it may present with failure to thrive.

Hypokalaemia and hyperchloraemia are associated with nephrolithiasis and nephrocalcinosis in this condition. There is a non-anion gap metabolic acidosis (anion gap = $Na + K - HCO_3 - Cl$). Normal anion gap is < 15.

4.6   (c), (e)

The most common type of CAH is the 21-hydroxylase deficiency. The genes for this condition have been localised to the short arm of chromosome 6. There is autosomal recessive transmittance. Prenatal diagnosis is possible using DNA probes for the affected gene. 17-OH-progesterone levels are elevated in amniotic fluid. This condition presents in females as a virilising condition, associated salt losing is found in around two thirds of these. In males, it may present as precocious puberty in childhood. Hypertension is a finding in 11-hydroxylase deficiency. Serum 17-OH-progesterone is elevated in the former.

4.7   (b), (c), (d), (e)

Lung compliance, defined as the pressure required to inflate the lung by unit volume, is reduced in bronchopulmonary dysplasia (BPD) and in RDS in preterm infants, the former due to extensive fibrosis and unevenly emphysematous areas of the lung and the latter owing to reduced surfactant. Bronchial reactivity is increased and bronchodilators are often needed in infancy. Local areas of hyperinflation are common in BPD. The role of inhaled (and nebulised steroids) is still being explored and is controversial – there is evidence that it is useful, although the long-term effects of this are not clear.

4.8   (a), (b), (d), (e)

4.9   None

Methaemoglobinaemia is a disorder in which there is conversion of the ferrous form of haemoglobin to a ferric state in the intact red cell. Cyanosis in the absence of respiratory and cardiac causes occurs and a low SpO_2 accompanies a normal PO_2. The blood does not redden on exposure and stays brown. Inherited forms of the disease present at birth or at 2–4 months of age, depending on the chains affected (γ or β). Aniline dyes, dapsone and nitrites are toxic causes for methaemoglobinaemia. In recent times, the use of inhaled nitric oxide in ventilation is a common cause for methaemoglobinaemia. In the toxic forms, treatment with methylene blue is used.

4.10   (b), (d)

Duchenne muscular dystrophy (DMD) presents with delayed walking by the age of 18 months, and is not a cause for a floppy baby (an example of a floppy baby – spinal muscular atrophy type 1). Speech delay and mental retardation are also seen. Gene probes are being increasingly used to diagnose and for genetic counselling and the role of a muscle biopsy to diagnose DMD is becoming less clear. The abnormal product is a muscle protein called dystrophin. Frame-shift mutations causing a useless protein form cause the severe form of the disease. In contrast, Becker dystrophy, which presents with similar features at a later age, is characterised by lesser amounts of the normal protein and is much less severe.

4.11   (b), (e)

Localised mastocytosis (in the form of urticaria pigmentosa) presents as hyperpigmented spots between 1 and 9 months of age, which may be pruritic and blister. In systemic mastocytosis, pruritus is generalised. The latter implies infiltration of mast cells all over the body including liver, spleen and bone. A list of drugs, such as aspirin, morphine, codeine, radiographic contrast media and procaine, are contraindicated because of their mast cell degranulatory effects.

4.12   (a), (c), (e)

In Wolf–Parkinson–White (WPW) syndrome, an accessory bundle (bundle of Kent) between the atria and the ventricle conducts impulses bypassing the AV node. However, in the normal state this only causes the characteristic short PR interval and delta wave on the resting ECG. As an arrythmia, it is characterised by forward conduction of impulses by the AV node and a backward conduction up the accessory bundle, causing a re-entry phenomenon. These complexes are narrow, regular and are controlled by intravenous adenosine. Verapamil is contraindicated.

4.13   (c), (d)

Early features of heart failure do not include cyanosis (it may be a symptom of the underlying problem *per se*, but as a symptom of cardiac failure occurs quite late), oedema (weight gain may be more relevant) or bradycardia (rather tachycardia). Features are very subtle in infancy and include sweating while feeding, intermittent feeding rather than in a continuous pattern and tachypnoea while feeding.

4.14   (a), (e)
Congenital toxoplasmosis presents with microcephaly, a small-for-gestational-age baby, intracranial calcifications, hydrocephalus, chorio-retinitis, hepatosplenomegaly, low platelets and anaemia, and eye problems including glaucoma. Sore throat and cervical lymph nodes as well as flu-like symptoms are part of the primary infection with *Toxoplasma*. This commonly occurs in adults and older children and resembles a mononucleosis-like illness. A history of exposure to cats is usually elicited.

4.15   (b), (d)
Median nerve injury in the antecubital fossa causes loss of flexion of the second phalanges of all fingers, terminal phalanges of the index and middle fingers, partial loss of pronation only due to intact brachioradialis, loss of abduction and flexion of the thumb and sensory loss over the radial three and a half fingers and the dorsal surfaces of the same fingers.

4.16   (c), (d), (e)
Rickets is a generalised disorder of bone metabolism, commonly due to nutritional or genetic causes. Nutritional vitamin D deficiency is common in malnutrition and presents with inadequate mineralisation of the bone osteoid. A radiograph of a growing long bone (like at the wrist) would show a large gap between the metaphysis and epiphysis, cupping, splaying and fraying of the metaphysis. Non-accidental injury usually causes fractures and bucket-handle tears of the epiphyses, but not a discrete bone lesion.

4.17   (c)
Iron is absorbed in the proximal small intestine aided by ascorbic acid and gastric fluid. Absorbed iron in the ferrous form is bound to transferrin and transported in the serum to the liver, renal and bone marrow cells where it is stored as ferritin after combination with apoferritin. Intestinal mucosal cells regulate the intake of iron from the diet (< 10% ingested iron is absorbed in the normal state) by the ratio of apoferritin and ferritin

in the cell. Ferritin is a form of iron storage from which iron can be extracted for use, haemosiderin is an irreversible form and does not contribute the convertible form of iron storage.

4.18   (b), (c)
Generalised absences are common in girls in the school age group and present with recurrent episodes of blank spells. Loss of tone is uncommon in typical absences and is more characteristic of atonic seizures seen in Lennox-Gastaut syndrome. The typical EEG findings of a 3/sec spike and wave activity is diagnostic and the diagnosis is doubtful if it is absent on several EEGs. Hyperventilation, sleep deprivation and photic stimulation are methods to uncover changes if the resting EEG is normal. Treatment with ethosuximide or sodium valproate is effective.

4.19   (a), (b)
An abnormal CFTR (transmembrane regulator) protein is responsible for CF and the commonest gene mutation in Caucasians is in the ΔF-508 gene segment on chromosome 15. The defect is therefore a gene defect. This defect results in a high level of Na^+ and Cl^- in sweat, a commonly used test in clinical practice to diagnose CF. Values of Na^+ and Cl^- > 60 mmol/l are diagnostic, between 50 mmol/l and 60 mmol/l are borderline and need repeating. It is important to make sure that at least 100 mg of sweat is obtained. Psuedo-Bartter syndrome is seen in CF due to excessive Na^+ loss in the sweat.

4.20   (c), (d), (e)

4.21   (c)
There is pulmonary oligaemia in tetralogy of Fallot (due to pulmonary stenosis) and in Eisenmenger's syndrome (due to high pulmonary vascular resistance). Coarctation of the aorta presents with rib notching due to collaterals if left undetected after the neonatal period. There is associated hypertension. *Pneumocystis carinii* infection causes pneumonia.

4.22   (a), (d), (e)

4.23   (b)

4.24   (c)

RSV bronchiolitis is a lethal disease in babies with poor cardiopulmonary reserve as in chronic lung disease and congenital heart disease. Ribavirin has been used in these infants to prevent severe complications and ventilation. RSV immunoglobulin has been tried but has not proved to be of benefit, partly because of concerns over the volume of infusion needed. Recently, a monoclonal antibody to RSV (palivizumab) has been tried, and in a trial (IMpact), a 55% reduction of hospitalisation in RSV bronchiolitis was seen. It is given as a series of intra-muscular injections during the RSV season (five in number). Controversy still surrounds its exact benefits. A post-bronchiolitic wheezy stage is recognised and seems to be commoner in children with an atopic family background.

4.25   (a), (e)

Brucellosis is called undulant fever and follows transmission of *Brucella* from animals (especially in unpasteurised milk or milk products as well as contact with animals). The clinical features are non-specific and consist of recurrent fever, malaise, arthralgia and depression. Hepatosplenomegaly is seen in half the cases. Prior to antibiotics, 75% blood culture positivity is seen. Tetracyclines with aminoglycosides in combination are effective treatment regimens. Weil's test is positive in typhus infection.

4.26   (a), (b), (c), (e)

Certain phage types of staphylococci are responsible for toxin-mediated disease. Scalded skin syndrome is seen with phage type 4 infection. An immune-mediated response is seen with toxic shock syndrome due to the toxin acting as a super-antigen and triggering an uncontrolled immune response.

4.27   (c), (d), (e)

4.28   (b), (c), (e)

4.29   (a), (d)

4.30   (a), (c)

The commonest reactions to starting carbamazepine are a pancytopenia, which may occur at any time during the treatment and abnormal liver functions. Other side effects include drowsiness and diplopia.

Section 5

5.1 (a), (b), (c)
Klinefelter's syndrome is characterised by the karyotype XXY, although there can be variants with more X chromosomes. It is rarely diagnosed before puberty, at which time the expected pubertal changes fail to appear. In childhood, this condition should be suspected in mental retardation and in psychosocial, learning and behavioural problems. It is a chromosomal anomaly and not a genetic condition. High levels of FSH/LH are common after the age of 10.

5.2 (a), (c), (e)
Morquio syndrome is a mucopolysaccharidosis with typical skeletal changes, without mental involvement, as opposed to Hurler and Hunter syndromes (type I and II mucopolysaccharidoses) in which mental retardation is common. It causes short stature due to truncal (vertebral) shortening, and the limb length is usually normal. Atlantoaxial dislocation is a life-threatening complication, and serial MRI scans are commonly done to assess this.

5.3 (a), (d)
Hereditary spherocytosis and HHT (Osler–Weber–Rendu syndrome) are autosomal dominant transmitted. In the latter there are multiple telangiectasias in the skin, mucosa and lungs (these may be the cause of a left to right shunt and cardiac failure). CAH and Wilson's disease are autosomal recessive transmitted. Hypophosphataemic rickets is X-linked dominant. It usually presents in infancy but may be delayed up to 5 years. Hyperphosphaturia is seen with a consequent hypophosphataemia. Treatment is with oral phosphates and alfacalcidol.

5.4 (a), (b), (c), (e)
Dubowitz criteria to assess gestational age employ physical criteria and neurological criteria to score infants. A cumulative score is then plotted on a graph to establish the gestational age. Popliteal angle and scarf sign are indicators of changing tone with gestational age, whereas Moro's reflex is a primitive neurological reflex that appears around 32 weeks gestation and disappears by 3 months.

5.5 (b), (e)

5.6 (a), (c), (e)

Acute graft-versus host (GVH) reaction occurs when an immuno-compromised individual has immunocompetent lymphocytes infused from another person, which act against host MHC antigens. It common-ly occurs within the first 100 days following a bone marrow transplant. Diarrhoea, liver involvement, rash, and a falling blood count suggest acute onset of GVH. Another instance of possible GVH is a premature neonate/immunocompromised child receiving non-irradiated blood (irradiation inactivates lymphocytes).

5.7 (a), (b), (e)

Growth hormone (GH) is being used to increase stature in Turner and Russell-Silver syndrome. Panhypopituitarism causes GH deficiency and is an indication to use GH. Craniopharyngioma by itself may not lead to short stature although the treatment, e.g. radiotherapy, might cause GH deficiency.

5.8 (a), (c)

Microangiopathic changes causing retinal changes, renal changes, and vascular/neurological changes are rare before the age of puberty, mainly because they take a few years of poorly controlled diabetes to cause problems. Although diabetes can be associated with other autoimmune conditions like Addison's disease and hyperthyroidism, it is not neces-sarily always true. Lumpy changes from lipodystrophy are common in the areas of injections and are reasons for poor control of diabetes due to poor absorption of the insulin from these sites. Isophane insulin (medium-term action) acts slower compared to plain insulin (quick action).

5.9 (a), (b). (c), (d)

5.10   (c), (e)

Most important in the acute management of asthma is giving O_2. An arterial blood gas is useless in guiding management in a child with acute severe asthma. Salbutamol is a β_2-agonist.

5.11 (a), (b), (d)

Electrolyte imbalance, cardiac failure and cardiac arrythmias are causes of death in anorexia and bulimia. Calluses on the hands from stimulation of vomiting by gagging are seen in bulimia. Like anorexia nervosa, this condition is common in girls. Most often bulimia is a *de novo* phenomenon, although in some it may follow anorexia. Eroded dental enamel, hypokalaemia and impaired renal function are common side effects. These patients tend to be slightly overweight or normal in weight.

5.12 (a), (d), (e)

Ebstein's anomaly is a cardiac disease with an abnormally positioned septal leaflet of the tricuspid valve. This commonly leads to gross tricuspid regurgitation and a right to left shunt through the patent foramen ovale. In a supradiaphragmatic TAPVD, all the pulmonary veins drain into the right atrium carrying oxygenated blood to the right side of the heart. This may give the appearance of a 'snow-man heart' with a bulge at the level of the SVC (superior vena cava) and then a large right atrium.

5.13 (b), (d), (e)

Haemoglobin (Hb) < 5 g% does not leave enough deoxygenated Hb to present clinically as cyanosis. Methaemoglobinaemia causes cyanosis but the PaO_2 is normal and the cyanosis does not get any better with O_2. The blood looks brown on exposure to air and does not turn red. R–L shunts, as in Eisenmenger complex, or as in TOF and TGA, will not respond to increases in O_2. Only pulmonary causes of cyanosis respond to O_2 therapy.

5.14 (a), (b), (d)

Intususception is a common surgical emergency in infancy and the second year of life, presenting classically with vomiting, intermittent colicky pain, red currant jelly stools, and a sausage-shaped mass in the abdomen. Management includes reduction with a contrast enema/air enema. Perforation/gangrene is an indication for open surgery as is an unstable child with cardiovascular compromise. Failed reduction is managed with open surgery.

5.15 (a), (c), (d)

Epstein–Barr virus (EBV) infection affects the B cells; however, the atypical lymphocytes and the other responses are T-cell mediated (CD8$^+$). Ampicillin or amoxicillin cause rashes with EBV infection.

5.16   (a), (c)

A 36-month old would ride a tricycle, repeat three digits, play with other children in simple play, help in dressing/undressing, and build a tower of 10 cubes. A 4-year old names four colours and indulges in symbolic play. At 3 years, a child can draw a man with a head and about two limbs.

5.17   (a), (b), (e)

5.18   (a), (c), (d), (e)

Herpangina is an infection of the fauces and pharynx, presenting with ulceration. Dermatitis herpetiformis is an immune-mediated skin condition, with no relation to herpes virus. It is treated with dapsone. Epidemic pleurodynia or Bornholm disease is an infection caused by coxsackie viruses, characterised by severe pleuritic pain in the chest.

5.19   (a), (c), (d)

Hand dominance, adductor spasm and the presence of neonatal reflexes like Moro or grasp indicate the diagnosis of cerebral palsy.

5.20   (c), (e)

5.21   (b), (d)

5.22   (a), (b), (c), (d)

Renal vein thrombosis presents classically with a loin mass and haematuria. It is seen usually in dehydrated infants, infants with polycythaemia, and in children with nephrotic syndrome. Conservative management is advised if the thrombus is unilateral and does not extend into the IVC (inferior vena cava). Thrombectomy/anticoagulation is advised in bilateral cases to prevent renal failure.

5.23   None

None of these choices favour a non-organic cause over an organic one. A long history does not necessarily mean a non-organic cause. In Crohn's disease, there may be a long history before the diagnosis is made and mouth ulcers may be associated with anal tags and fissures. A family history of peptic ulcer disease and migraine may favour an ulcer or abdominal migraine, respectively.

5.24   (c)
Shigella, Salmonella and *Campylobacter* are all causes of bloody diarrhoea. *Giardia* infection causes recurrent or chronic diarrhoea with mal-absorption and dyspepsia.

5.25   (a), (b), (c)
Galactosaemia is an inherited disorder of galactose metabolism in which there is an absence of the enzyme galactose-1-phosphate uridyl trans-ferase. Affected infants present within days after ingesting milk (especially breast milk) and develop failure to thrive, diarrhoea, liver failure and sepsis with Gram-negative organisms. Cataracts develop soon after birth. Hypoglycaemia is common in affected infants. Complete elimination of galactose from the diet prevents the early complications and mortality. However, the long-term complications like visual perception and intellectual dysfunction as well as sterility in females is not prevented even with a rigorous dietary schedule.

5.26   (a), (b), (c), (e)
Although *Mycoplasma* infection is best known to cause respiratory symptoms, it can cause bullous myringitis, cardiac conduction problems, neurological sequelae like Guillan–Barré syndrome, skin changes as in Stevens-Johnson syndrome, haemolytic anaemia and low platelets.

5.27   (b), (d), (e)
Umbilical hernia is commoner in premature babies, hypothyroid infants, in mucopolysaccharidoses, and in black children. Most defects close by the age of 3–4 years, and only the obstructed ones or those that increase in size after 2 years need surgery.

5.28   (b), (e)

5.29   (a), (d), (e)
ABO incompatibility arises from antibodies to A or B antigens on the foetus from the mother who is usually of blood group O. This can occur in the first pregnancy, and can present with a weak or negative Coombs test due to incomplete antibodies.

5.30   (b), (c), (d), (e)

Section 6

6.1 None

The commonest mutation in Caucasians causing CF is the ΔF-508. The prevalence of this mutation in the general population is around 1/25. More than 100 mutations have been described for the disease and prenatal testing is impossible for all cases. The affected protein is called the CFTR protein (it is a trans-membrane chloride channel). There does not seem to be a strict correlation between the phenotype and the genotype in CF. Some genotypes present with mild disease and some with severe disease. The organs affected are the lungs, pancreas, skin sweat glands, seminiferous tubules and fallopian tubes. Complications include respiratory disease with bronchiectasis, failure to thrive with steatorrhoea, meconium ileus in neonates, diabetes mellitus, infertility and pseudo-Barrtter syndrome.

6.2 (a), (c), (e)

Although each clinical setting dictates its own plan, thyroid functions and urine culture are easily done and are necessary in the workup of a child with failure to thrive. A sweat test is trickier, and is done more often than not in clinical practice. Colonoscopy and jejunal biopsy are invasive procedures reserved for cases with good clinical history of malabsorption from Crohn's or coeliac disease.

6.3   None

Chronic carrier of hepatitis B will not manifest any clinical or biochemical signs, and only testing for HBsAg will be diagnostic. Antenatal testing is mandatory and if a mother is found positive in pregnancy, the newborn infant definitely needs the recombinant hepatitis B vaccine given at 0, 1 and 3 months. Additionally, hepatitis B immunoglobulin is also given at the same time if the Hep BeAg is positive (this is an indicator of infectivity), the status is unknown, is doubtful or there are no anti-HBe antibodies in the serum. There is a strong case for universal vaccination with HB vaccine as is practised in the US.

6.4 (a), (e)

The commonest drugs used to control seizures in children are sodium valproate and carbamazepine. Phenytoin causes serious side effects including gingival hypertrophy, hirsutism, cerebellar signs, rickets and pseudolymphomas – all of which are undesirable in a child. Lamotrigine is commonly used as an adjunctive drug although it is being used infrequently as monotherapy. Topiramate is also used rarely as adjunctive therapy, primarily in intractable seizures or seizures difficult to control on common drugs.

6.5   (a), (c)

An INR at this range is accompanied by serious bleeding problems and is best treated by giving fresh-frozen plasma. Cryoprecipitate is a rich source of factors involved in the intrinsic pathway like VIII, IX and is used in haemophilia and von Willebrand's disease (vWD). Vitamin K is useful to reverse the antagonism of warfarin. Tranexamic acid is an antifibrinolytic and can be used in haemophilia and vWD (as is desmopressin which releases the factor into the blood transiently).

6.6   (a), (b), (c)

Long term TPN for > 4 weeks is associated with problems with trace metal deficiency such as Zn, Mn, Se, Fe and Cu. Calcium and phosphate are essential elements and should be normal constituents of TPN. Regular serum Na, K, Ca, PO_4, urea, creatinine, LFTs (liver-function tests) and Mg are needed prior to the 4 weeks.

6.7   (a), (d), (e)

Hypogonadism can be associated with low FSH and LH (hypogonadotropic) as in Kallman syndrome (anosmia and hypogonadism), Prader–Willi syndrome, Bardet Biedl syndrome or with high levels of FSH and LH (hypergonadotropic) as in testicular atrophy, Klinefelter syndrome and Noonan syndrome.

6.8   (b), (c), (d)

Steroids in doses such as this do not cause lasting effects on growth to cause short stature. Osteogenesis imperfecta is associated with fractures and may lead to short stature. Morquio syndrome is a mucopolysaccharidosis, which is typified by truncal shortening and normal limb size and normal intellect, in contrast to hypochondroplasia, which has normal truncal proportions and short limbs (milder form of achondroplasia). 11β-OH deficiency causes CAH and leads to a virilised female with hypertension (as a result of the elevated levels of deoxycortisone).

6.9   (a), (c)

Recurrent haematuria is distinct from acute post-streptococcal nephritis. The common causes are IgA nephropathy (Berger's nephropathy) and renal stones. Alport syndrome is an X-linked disease with familial or hereditary nephritis and deafness, but is uncommon. IgA nephritis presents as a first episode of gross haematuria soon after a viral infection (2–4 days as opposed to 1–2 weeks in acute post-streptococcal disease) and then settles down (a phase of microscopic haematuria) only to recur with another viral infection. Deposits of IgA are found in mesangial deposits. Prognosis is in general good, but around 30% will develop progressive disease and are treated with immunosuppressive drugs. Prognosis in childhood may be better than in adults.

6.10   (a), (b), (c), (e)

Hepatitis B vaccine is given as an intramuscular injection.

6.11   (c), (e)

Packed cell transfusions (not whole blood!) with desferrioxamine (for iron chelation to prevent iron overload and haemochromatosis), and a bone marrow transplant are the treatment options in β-thalassaemia. Pneumovax and prophylactic penicillin are important in hyposplenic individuals like sickle cell patients or those who have had a splenectomy.

6.12   (a)

TOF and tricuspid atresia are cyanotic heart diseases with reduced pulmonary flow. Tricuspid regurgitation and Eisenmenger syndrome are a result of pulmonary hypertension, not causes.

6.13   (a), (b), (c), (d)

Common causes for recurrent headaches in childhood include migraine (both typical and atypical), tension headaches, refractive errors, sinusitis and referred pain from earache. An MRI scan may be needed in headaches with persisting visual problems, deteriorating school performance, amblyopic attacks, lateralising neurological signs, behavioural changes, cough headache and early morning headaches. Uncommon but important causes for headaches include CO poisoning and lead poisoning, benign intracranial hypertension and chronic subdural haematoma.

6.14 (a), (c), (d)

Foetal distress is indicated by type II decelerations on the CTG, which are slow to recover and start coming back to the baseline after the peak of the uterine contraction. Type I decelerations are normal responses *in utero* to the uterine pressure on the foetal head and are manifested by quick return to the baseline just after the peak of the uterine contraction. Arrhythmias are not usually indicative of foetal distress, rather suggesting an underlying heart problem. Meconium staining has been recognised as a sign of intrauterine hypoxia, especially when it is thick and 'pea soup' type.

6.15 (a), (c), (e)

Bit of controversy here! The only curative mode for a SCID is a bone marrow transplant (BMT) and therefore although SCID is not very common, it is common to do a BMT on these children. Acute lymphoblastic leukemia, on the other hand, is treated with chemotherapy in about 70% and the indication for a BMT is in high-risk groups such as infants, WBC > 100,000/mm^3, failure to achieve remission, relapse on chemotherapy or after the second relapse. Gaucher's disease is uncommon. Aplastic anaemia is an indication for a BMT.

6.16 (b), (c), (e)

Curosurf is a natural surfactant from porcine lungs. Antenatal steroids are given intramuscularly 12 hours apart. Either dexamethasone or betamethasone are used and for maximum benefit should be given at least 12 hours prior to delivery. They need to be repeated after a week if preterm delivery is still imminent. Mean airway pressure (MAP) is influenced most by a change in PEEP (positive end-expiratory pressure). Other factors include PIP (peak inspiratory pressure) and inspiratory time. MAP is the chief determinant of oxygenation. Rate affects the minute ventilation and therefore CO_2 elimination. Pressure–volume curves shift to the right with surfactant (increased compliance of the lung).

6.17 (c), (e)

Addison's disease is an autoimmune condition and is often part of an autoimmune polyendocrinopathy. Type I is Addison's with chronic mucocutaneous candidiasis or hypoparathyroidism or alopecia or vitiligo or chronic active hepatitis or insulin-dependent diabetes mellitus (IDDM) or hypothyroidism. Type II is with IDDM or thyroid disease.

6.18   (a), (c)
Anaemia and jaundice are common in severe malaria.

6.19   (a)
For more details on the complement pathway, refer to Forfar and Arneil's *Textbook of Paediatrics,* London: Churchill Livingstone, 5th edn, p. 1234.

6.20   (a), (d), (e)
Secretory diarrhoea is caused by active secretion of fluid and ions into the gut lumen as in cholera, entero-toxigenic *E. coli* infection, chloridorrhoea and VIPoma (vasoactive intestinal peptide). Osmotic diarrhoea, on the other hand, is caused by the osmotically active ions/products as in lactose intolerance (lactose), CF (malabsorption from pancreatic deficiency and undigested food), blind loop syndrome (osmotic particles by bacterial degradation), etc.

6.21   (a), (b), (d)
Reye syndrome is an encephalopathy as is Leigh disease. The latter consists of at least three types: deficient pyruvate dehydrogenase complex, deficient complex I, or deficient complex IV of the respiratory chain. Infants have feeding problems, vomiting, failure to thrive, seizures, hypotonia, nystagmus and pyramidal signs. Elevated serum lactate levels are characteristic. Canavan disease is an autosomal recessive transmitted disorder with spongy degeneration of the white matter presenting as progressive macrocephaly, persistent head lag and hypotonia at around 3–6 months of age. High levels of *N*-acetyl aspartate are found in urine, blood and CSF.

6.22   (c)
Although choices (a), (b) and (c) are causes for respiratory distress at birth, RDS is the commonest. Meconium aspiration is uncommon with better management of the infant born through meconium. Choices (d) and (e) do not cause respiratory distress.

6.23   (a), (e)
The British Thoracic Society guidelines for the management of asthma from *Thorax,* **52** (Suppl 1), February, 1997, S1–S20, suggest the accepted lines of managing asthma. Montelucast is a new leucotriene receptor antagonist, which is being used for chronic asthma. There has not been

enough accumulated evidence to support its use in routine clinical practice. Suggested step where it may be added onto treatment: in moderate chronic asthma after inhaled corticosteroids (to enable a reduction in dosage of steroid).

6.24   (a), (b), (e)

All these cause seizures in a neonate, but pyridoxine deficiency and hydrocephalus are rare in everyday practice. Hypomagnesaemia can also cause seizures.

6.25   (d)

Toddler's diarrhoea is a benign cause of recurrent or chronic diarrhoea in the age range of 1–3 years. It is not associated with failure to thrive. It may form part of the spectrum of disorders ranging from infantile colic, irritable bowel to recurrent abdominal pain. Food intolerance and post-enteritis diarrhoea are the chief differential diagnoses.

6.26   (a), (b), (c), (d), (e)

Injury to the VII nerve at the stylomastoid foramen causes a lower motor neuron palsy on the same side with inability to close the eyes, loss of sensation from the anterior third of the tongue due to lingual nerve damage and no sensory loss on the face (supplied by V nerve). The chorda tympani nerve supplies the taste sensation for the anterior third of the tongue and exits before the stylomastoid foramen.

6.27   (a), (c), (e)

The bacteriology of sputum in CF changes from *Staphylococcus aureus* (in infancy) to *Haemophilus* to *Pseudomonas* (in childhood). *Burkholderia* was formerly *Pseudomonas cepacia* and is not common, but when it is present indicates rapid deterioration of respiratory function and cor pulmonale.

6.28   (a), (b), (d)

6.29   (a), (d), (e)

Child abuse can take various forms and is often very difficult to diagnose. The four main categories include physical, sexual and emotional abuse, and neglect. Suspicious signs of physical abuse include large bruises in a child who is relatively immobile like an infant, multiple bruises of varying ages in uncommon areas, characteristic signs like bite marks or cigarette burns, posterior rib fractures on chest radiographs and patterned bruises like hot plate injury to the buttocks. Sexual abuse is suspected if a child indulges in inappropriate sexual play, is sexually aggressive to other children, refuses to stay with some well known and familiar person in the recent past or if there is vaginal bleeding/discharge in a young child.

6.30   (b), (e)

Still's disease (or systemic juvenile chronic arthritis) manifests with fever, splenomegaly and rash, and is sometimes accompanied by joint symptoms. By definition, the time scale of juvenile chronic arthritis is in weeks (6 weeks for a diagnosis) rather than in days. The classification is as follows: systemic onset, polyarticular and pauciarticular types. The pauciarticular type is the commonest and is associated with uveitis. It occurs in two distinct groups – younger girls (antinuclear factor positive) and older boys. The polyarticular type is the type most akin to adult RA (rheumatoid factor positive) in some of the cases.

Section 7

7.1 (a), (b), (c), (d), (e)

Homocystinuria is an autosomal recessive inherited disease affecting the metabolic pathway of methionine. The commonest type, type I, is due to a deficient enzyme, cystathionine synthase, which leads to accumulation of homocystine just proximal to the defect. Features include marfanoid features, dislocation of the lens downward and inwards, recurrent thromboembolic phenomena, mental retardation and psychiatric changes. High doses of vitamin B_6 produce good improvements in patients who respond to it; supplemental folate therapy, restricted methionine intake and betaine (which lowers levels of homocystine in the body) are useful adjuncts.

7.2 (a), (c)

Pre-ductal coarctation of the aorta is common in Turner's syndrome. This is usually the cause for hypertension in this disorder, although hypertension may occur without it. The presence of femoral pulses does not rule out the coarctation. Associations include intracranial aneurysms and bicuspid aortic valve. The commonest heart lesion is a VSD.

7.3 (a), (e)

7.4 (c), (d)

Mortality from asthma has not changed in the UK in the last 5 years, even though there is now better recognition and better treatment of asthma. Nocturnal cough may be the only symptom in children. RSV bronchiolitis causes wheezing with URTIs in atopically predisposed children.

7.5 (a), (d), (e)

Ceftazidime can be used with caution.

7.6 (a), (d)

The ulnar nerve supplies all the muscles of the hypothenar eminence and the adductor pollicis from the thenar group. Sensory supply of the forearm proximal to the wrist is from the medial cutaneous nerve of the forearm from the brachial plexus.

7.7 (a), (d), (e)
The differentiation between a lower motor neuron (LMN) and an upper motor neuron (UMN) facial palsy is by the involvement of the upper half of the face in an LMN-type lesion.

7.8 (b), (d)
Insulin-like growth factor (IGF) is a single chain polypeptide released from the liver from growth hormone (GH). The bodily effects of GH are mediated by the IGF, which circulates in blood bound to somatomedin binding protein. GH is released in a pulsatile fashion when measured by radio-immunoassay (RIA) but there is evidence that it is more rhythmic than pulsatile when measured by RIMA (radioimmunometric assay).

7.9 (a), (c), (d)
An abnormal CFTR (transmembrane regulator) protein is responsible for CF and the commonest gene mutation in Caucasians is in the ΔF-508 gene segment on chromosome 15. The defect is therefore a gene defect. This defect results in a high level of Na and Cl in sweat, a commonly used test in clinical practice to diagnose CF. Values of Na and Cl > 60 mmol/l are diagnostic, between 50 mmol/l and 60 mmol/l are borderline and need repeating. It is important to make sure that at least 100 mg of sweat is obtained.

7.10   (a), (b), (c), (d), (e)

7.11   (a), (b), (c)
Adverse effects of non-steroidal anti-inflammatory drugs (NSAIDs) include gastritis, renal papillary necrosis, reduced platelet function, fluid retention and renal impairment.

7.12   (b), (d), (e)
The keyword is diagnostic. C-reactive protein (C-RP) will only indicate inflammation; low C3 may be a feature of some diseases causing arthritis. Synovial fluid analysis indicates the diagnosis in infective and inflammatory conditions like rheumatoid arthritis (RA). In acute septic arthritis,

there is a polymorphonuclear predominance and elevated protein levels. The factor IX assay is useful in a child with a haemarthrosis from haemophilia B.

7.13   (a), (d)
Serum C3 levels are normal in Henoch–Schoenlein purpura and in haemolytic uraemic syndrome. Type II mesangiocapillary glomerulo-nephritis is characterised by mesangial deposition of C3. Systemic lupus erythematosus (SLE) is diagnosed by the presence of anti-nuclear antibods, especially anti-double stranded DNA, which correlates with renal disease.

7.14   (e)
CVID is a term for a heterogenous group of immune disorders that involve predominant defects in B cells and no defects in T cells. In Bruton's agammaglobulinaemia, the lack of B cells is absolute. IgA levels may not be normal. Association with other autoimmune disorders is seen, but no specific inheritance pattern is identified.

7.15   (a), (b)
Conditions that cause an increased left-ventricular end diastolic volume (LVEDV) result in a volume overload on the heart and therefore follow left-sided regurgitant lesions. In congestive cardiomyopathy, there is hypofunction of most of the myocardium. Common causes of the same finding in adults would be ischaemia of the LV myocardium. A pericardial effusion would cause restricted inflow of blood to the heart.

7.16   (a), (c), (e)
The features of constrictive pericarditis include gradual onset of dyspnoea, ascites, pulsatile liver, distended neck veins, narrow pulses, quiet precordium, faint pericardial rub, pericardial knock and normal liver functions. Causes include post-irradiation, TB, postviral pericarditis, purulent pericarditis and neoplastic infiltration of the pericardium.

7.17   (a), (b), (e)
FISH is fluorescent in-situ hybridisation. It is useful in diagnosing minor abnormalities in chromosomes that do not show up on normal karyotyping. The 22q11 deletion in DiGeorge is thus clearly identified by this technique. It involves attaching a fluorescent dye to a complementary

strand of DNA (to the area of interest) and looking for the dye by fluorescence when hybridised with the sample to be tested. Absent areas will not fluoresce. In Prader–Willi and Angelman syndromes, the area of interest is chromosome 15 q12.

7.18   (a), (b), (c), (d)
Renal concentration mechanisms are not fully developed even in term neonates and there may be elevated renal sodium losses in the initial phase of life. The presence of only two vessels in the cord may signify an associated renal anomaly and therefore, renal ultrasound scans are needed in any neonate identified to have the problem.

7.19   (a), (c), (e)
The differentiation of EHBA (extrahepatic biliary atresia) from neonatal hepatitis in a child with cholestasis is often difficult. A combination of clinical, radiological and biochemical tests will help. Hepatomegaly, persistently acholic stools, associated polysplenia or other intra-abdominal vascular anomalies, normal uptake on a HIDA scan with no excretion, liver biopsy suggestive of periportal fibrosis and oedema with bile ductular proliferation and bile plugs are all supportive of EHBA. Neonatal hepatitis is familial in 20% cases and the liver biopsy shows destruction of the architecture of the liver and marked inflammatory cell infiltrate.

7.20   (a)
In paediatric cardiac arrest, hypoxia is the main culprit. Cardiac causes as seen in adults is very rare, except in cardiac units. For this reason, asystole is more common than ventricular fibrillation as a rhythm at presentation. Intracardiac adrenaline is no longer used routinely. The ratio of compressions and respirations is 15:2 in this age group. Calcium is only given in documented hypocalcaemia.

7.21   (a), (d), (e)

7.22   (a), (c), (e)

7.23   (a), (b), (c), (d), (e)
Except in a cleft palate, the cause for deafness is sensorineural. In the child with a cleft palate, Eustachian tube dysfunction causes serous otitis with conductive deafness. Alport syndrome is a hereditary disease (X-

linked) with nephritis, renal failure and deafness. Deafness from meningitis is probably immunological and dexamethasone is given in most cases to avoid this complication (evidence for preventing *Haemophilus* infection-related deafness is strong).

7.24   (a), (b), (c), (e)
Peak expiratory flow rate (PEFR) is a sensitive measurement of small airway obstruction, although the maximal mid-expiratory flow rate is more altered in mild disease. The ease of performing the PEFR at the bedside has made it more relevant in clinical practice. It changes more with height than age, and is effort independent if proper technique is used.

7.25   (b), (d)
Normal anion gap, growth failure, hyperventilation, and systemic acidosis are features of both the types. Type I or distal type is severe and is due to improper acidification of urine in the distal tubule. The urine pH will not lower below 5.5, even with maximal acid load. Nephrocalcinosis is a feature. Type II or proximal type is due to HCO_3 loss from the tubules and commonly forms part of syndromes such as the Fanconi's syndrome or Wilson's disease.

7.26   (a), (b), (c)

7.27   (b), (c), (d)
These features are part of *Toxoplasma* infection in humans. Chorioretinitis and microcephaly are seen with congenital infection. Affected infants present with intracerebral calcification in the periventricular area. Hydrocephalus, microcephaly, liver failure, thrombocytopenia and hepatosplenomegaly may also be seen. A mononucleosis-like syndrome is seen with acquired *Toxoplasma* infection consisting of lymphadenopathy, fever, malaise and atypical lymphocytes in the blood.

7.28   (a), (e)
All the others cause metaphyseal changes. In rickets, there is an increased gap between the metaphysis and the epiphysis due to unmineralised osteoid. There is also cupping, splaying and fraying of the metaphyseal end. Treatment in nutritional rickets results in rapid

healing and a line of mineralisation is obvious. Conradi syndrome is part of the spectrum of chondrodysplasia punctata, presenting with stippled epiphyses on radiographs.

7.29   (b), (c)

Renal osteodystrophy is caused by a multitude of factors including retention of phosphate, secondary hyperparathyroidism due to vitamin D deficiency and low calcium levels, intestinal malabsorption of calcium and abnormal vitamin D metabolism. Severity is determined by age at onset and duration of renal impairment. Clinically, it manifests at a GFR level below $25\,\mathrm{ml/min/1.73\,m^2}$. Poor growth, bone pain, slipped epiphyses and deformities result.

7.30   (a), (b), (e)

Section 8

8.1 (a), (e)
Antibodies found in various diseases include antiendomysial and anti-reticulin and antigliadin antibodies in coeliac disease, thyroid-stimulating hormone (TSH) receptor stimulating antibodies in Graves' disease, anti-neuromuscular junction antibodies in myasthenia gravis, islet cell antibodies in insulin-dependent diabetes mellitus (IDDM), anti-melanocyte antibodies in vitiligo, dsDNA and antihistone antibodies in SLE and specific antibodies like SS1 and SS2 in systemic sclerosis.

8.2 (a), (d)
Genetic anticipation refers to the increase in disease severity in successive generations, commonly seen in diseases like Huntington's chorea, myotonic dystrophy, Fragile X syndrome and Freidrich's ataxia, where there is an expansion of the tri-nucleotide repeat sequence with each generation. In myotonic dystrophy, an affected mother may have very few symptoms (myotonia when hand is shaken) but the affected infant has severe muscle weakness and may need ventilation in the neonatal period.

8.3 (b)
Hurler syndrome presents with corneal clouding as opposed to opacities, which may be a result of corneal ulcers from past herpetic infection.

8.4 (b), (e)
Lymphoma is usually a complication of coeliac disease rather than a cause of malabsorption. Jejunal diverticula may be blind loops and predispose to bacterial overgrowth. *Giardia* infection causes acute symptoms of gastro-enteritis in some patients, but the commoner presentation is with chronic diarrhoea and failure to thrive. Diagnosis may be difficult and a fresh stool sample may show the trophozoites (repeated sampling is necessary in most instances due to the intermittent excretion). A duodenal aspirate is needed in extreme cases to confirm the diagnosis. Treatment with metronidazole is curative. Tinidazole is an alternative.

8.5 (e)

Infants with folate deficiency have failure to thrive, weakness and susceptibility to infections. In most such cases, a red cell folate tends to be lower than 160 ng/ml. Laboratory features may include macrocytosis and hypersegmented neutrophils. High-risk groups for deficiency states include premature infants who are not supplemented with folate, children with haemolytic anaemias and those with malabsorption.

8.6 (a), (c), (e)

Hepatitis C is borne by blood products as well as transmitted by sexual contact similar to hepatitis B.

8.7 (a), (b), (c)

The primary immunisation schedule of 2, 3, 4 months for HiB vaccine, DTP and OPV plus the 12–18-month MMR will render protection against these diseases. This is the immunisation schedule in UK. Babies born to Asian/African parents would also receive the BCG at birth. Pneumococcal vaccination is only given to children with hyposplenism.

8.8 (a), (b), (c)

In a normal distribution curve, the median and mean are the same. In a skewed curve, they may be different depending on the range of variables. Choice (d) pertains to prevalence not incidence. The lower the p value, the lower the possibility that the result is due to pure chance.

8.9 (a), (b)

Anion gap is calculated by the equation: $Na + K - HCO_3 - Cl$. This represents the unmeasured anions. In the presence of acidic products in the circulation, this value is raised, as in diabetic ketoacidosis (ketones) and shock (lactate). Thus, the causes of an increased anion gap include dehydration and lactic acidosis, DKA (diabetic ketoacidosis), alcoholic ketoacidosis and uraemia due to raised inorganic acids. Renal tubular causes usually cause normal anion gap acidosis due to a compensatory hyperchloraemia.

8.10 (b), (c), (d)
In many cases, unconjugated bilirubin levels are raised by an uncertain mechanism. Paradoxical aciduria in pyloric stenosis is an effort to concentrate sodium and maintain normovolaemia in preference to excreting alkali – the exchange mechanism of H^+–Na^+–K^+ acts here. A test feed being positive is sufficient clinical evidence that there is a pyloric obstruction and an ultrasound may confirm it. Barium swallow is not used routinely. It may have a role in very equivocal cases or when an ultrasound is not available.

8.11 (a), (b), (c), (d)

8.12 (a), (c)
Stroke may be a complication of a right to left shunt and the poly-cythaemia that accompanies it. In this situation, an infarction from venous thrombosis is common. Stroke is a rare but important complication of vasculitides like systemic lupus erythematosus (SLE). (For other causes of stroke, see Forfar and Arneil's *Textbook of Paediatrics*, London: Churchill Livingstone, 5th edn, p. 712.)

8.13 None
All are normal phenomena at the preschool age.

8.14 (b), (c)
The commonest cause of intrauterine growth retardation (IUGR) in the UK is not nutritional. Pre-eclampsia may be a risk factor. Other causes may consist of chromosomal disorders, intrauterine infections and maternal smoking and drug abuse. Although a lot of work continues in the role of growth hormone (GH) and IGF in IUGR, no clear deficiency has been demonstrated in foetuses or in later life.

8.15 (a), (c), (d)
Benign rolandic epilepsy (with centrotemporal spikes on the EEG) is a benign form of epilepsy with a peak age of occurrence at 8–10 years. It usually resolves by the age of 14–16 years, and is not treated unless it is recurrent or troublesome. The fits are focal, with involvement of the face and mouth (sometimes the upper limbs), and occur in sleep or in a drowsy state. Treatment with carbamazepine is usually fruitful.

8.16   (c)

Febrile convulsions are common between the ages of 6 months and 5 years, roughly affecting 1 in 20 children. It follows an infection and fever, and is typically a generalised seizure lasting less than 15 minutes, with full neurological recovery after the episode. Recurrence is common in 30% and is associated with a family history of fits or febrile fits. Atypical febrile convulsions may occur especially in children with neuro-developmental delay and may necessitate an EEG.

8.17   (b), (d)

Intussusception is common in infants, presents with sudden onset colicky abdominal pain, vomiting, passing 'red currant' jelly stools and examination reveals a pale child with intermittent colic, sometimes a lump in the abdomen and blood on per rectal exam. It can be acute, recurrent or chronic. It can be ileocolic (common), ileocolocolic, colocolic or ileoileal. Diagnostic investigations would include abdominal X-ray, ultrasound and a barium enema. Reduction is achieved by the enema itself – either barium or pneumatic. Henoch–Schoenlein purpura may present with an acute intussusception due to oedema and haemorrhage into the bowel wall.

8.18   (c), (e)

Acute laryngotracheobronchitis is usually caused by viruses – parainfluenza types 1 and 2, RSV and adenovirus – and is usually characterised by stridor (mostly inspiratory) and varying degrees of upper airway compromise. Nebulised adrenaline may be very helpful in the acute situation by reducing the airway oedema, although there is a risk of further rebound oedema after some time. Oral or nebulised steroids, mainly dexamethasone, have been found to be useful in many trials. Nebulised budesonide is also found to be effective in a dose of 2 mg given once or a divided dose of 1 mg twice. Supportive management is with oxygen as needed and feeding support.

8.19   (a), (b), (d), (e)

Sarcoptes scabeii is a mite, which infests only human hosts and causes scabies. The mite is seen in burrows in the interdigital spaces, but is difficult to demonstrate. Pruritus is a prominent symptom of scabies and may persist after treatment; it is mediated by a type IV hypersensitivity reaction. Although the common presentation is as papules, it can present as nodules (especially on the scrotum) or vesicles. Treatment is aimed at the whole family and comprises permethrin/malathion/benzyl benzoate.

8.20   (b), (c), (e)

8.21   (a), (b), (d)

8.22   (a)
Primidone and cyclosporine are the other drugs that cause gingival hypertrophy.

8.23   (b), (c), (d), (e)
Haemoglobin F is elevated in many disorders including thalassaemia, Fanconi's anaemia, sickle cell disease and some haemolytic anaemias such as hereditary spherocytosis. Persistence of haemoglobin F levels in infancy is seen in thalassaemia trait.

8.24   (a), (c), (d), (e)
Anorexia nervosa is characterised by an intense fear of being obese (even when underweight), distorted body image, weight < 15% of the expected percentile and amenorrhoea. Lowered mood, poor concentration and pre-occupation with food result from starvation. Although glucagon-like peptides are implicated, social factors play a vital role. A low bone marrow ratio, hypothyroidism and hypocortisolaemia, early osteopenia, bone marrow suppression, infections, low albumin levels, raised LFTs, hypokalaemia, hypoglycaemia and sensory peripheral neuropathy may complicate the condition.

8.25   (a), (e)

8.26   None
Renin is secreted in the juxtaglomerular apparatus in response to decreased filtrate in the glomerulus, indicating hypovolaemia and low renal perfusion. This then converts angiotensinogen into angiotensin I. This latter product is then converted into angiotensin II (AT II) by ACE, found in abundance in the pulmonary vessels. AT II is a potent vasoconstrictor and causes increased peripheral resistance to raise blood pressure. It also acts on aldosterone to increase sodium reabsorption in the late distal collecting tube (DCT) and collecting ducts.

8.27   (e)

Reflex anoxic seizures are benign episodes triggered by minor painful trauma in children of the preschool age group, although it may persist into adolescence. They are also variously called pallid breath holding spells and white breath holding spells. After a sudden collapse, there may be a brief period of twitching movements and then rapid recovery. It is usually not treated. Prognosis is excellent. No long-term neurological sequelae have been reported.

8.28   (b)

ITP is an immune-mediated disease with destruction of platelets by antibodies. It may occur as an acute form following a viral infection or as a chronic form (> 6 months). Prognosis in the acute form is good. Patients usually present with petechiae or bruising. Splenomegaly is not a feature, and its presence should alert one to another diagnosis, especially leukaemia. Treatment modalities range from just observation to oral steroids to intravenous immunoglobulin (reserved for ongoing mucosal bleeds or intracranial bleeding). In the chronic form, splenectomy is sometimes indicated.

8.29   (a), (b), (c)

Exchange transfusions are done in haemolytic disease of the newborn with Rh or ABO incompatibility. Acute chest syndrome in sickle cell disease is an indication for an exchange to lower the haemoglobin (Hb) S < 30%. Other such indications include priapism, stroke, severe vaso-occlusive crisis and prophylactic (to keep the Hb S < 30% in past stroke).

8.30   (b), (e)

The answer to this question assumes that *Shigella* dysentery is rare in the UK. Crohn's disease, *Campylobacter* infection and enterotoxigenic *E. coli* (ETEC) infection are commoner causes of bloody diarrhoea; gastrointestinal bleeding from Peutz–Jegher's syndrome (oral pigmentation and intestinal polyps) is rare.

Section 9

9.1 (a), (c), (e)

Mitochondrial DNA is transmitted from mother to child (sperm is deficient in mitochondrial DNA). The genome in the mitochondrial DNA is different from the normal nuclear DNA. Examples of mitochondrial DNA transmitted diseases include Leber's hereditary optic neuritis, MERRF (myoclonic epilepsy with ragged red fibres), MELAS (mitochondrial myopathy, encephalopathy, lactic acidosis and stroke-like episodes), Kearns Sayre syndrome and Pearson bone marrow–pancreas syndrome.

9.2 (a), (d), (e)

Marfan syndrome is an autosomal dominant inherited disease. There is increased limb length and arachnodactyly. Eye anomalies include ectopia lentis and myopia. Mitral valve prolapse, aortic regurgitation and dissecting aneurysms are seen. Cognitive impairment is seen in homocystinuria, not in Marfan's.

9.3 (a), (b)

9.4 (a), (e)

DMD is a muscular dystrophy, which presents with delayed walking beyond 18 months and calf pseudohypertrophy. Gower sign is positive due to weakness of proximal muscle at hips. Features similar to those in DMD may present later on in life in Becker dystrophy. Both are defects in the dystrophin gene – DMD is characterised by a total lack of functional dystrophin, Becker with decreased amounts of the protein. Frontal baldness and cataracts are seen in myotonic dystrophy. Diagnoses to consider in a floppy infant include spinal muscular atrophy, Down's syndrome, Prader–Willi syndrome and other metabolic disorders.

9.5 (b), (d)

HANE is transmitted by autosomal dominant inheritance. There is deficient activity of C1 esterase inhibitor and a low C4 and C2 as a result of uninhibited activity of complement. This causes angioedema, which may be in the gut and present as abdominal pain, but commonly presents as recurrent swelling at sites of trauma. Danazol has been used in the chronic phase of management. In the acute phase, FFP (fresh frozen plasma) or C1 esterase inhibitor concentrate is used to restore normal levels of the protein.

9.6 (a), (b)

Sumatriptan is a selective 5-HT$_1$ antagonist used in migraine in the acute phase. It acts in both classical and common migraine as well as in cluster headaches. Used either orally or subcutaneously, it causes side effects like flushing, hypotension, chest pain and arrythmias. Pizotifen, which is a serotonin antagonist, is used in prophylaxis of migraine.

9.7 (a), (c), (d)

9.8 None

None of the diseases are common in infancy. The question is not 'diseases which commonly present as rash' in infancy.

9.9 (a), (b), (d), (e)

Brucellosis is called undulant fever and follows transmission of *Brucella* from animals (especially unpasteurised milk or milk products as well as contact with animals). The clinical features are non-specific and consist of recurrent fever, malaise, arthralgia and depression. Hepatosplenomegaly is seen in half the cases. Prior to antibiotics, 75% blood culture positivity is seen. A combination of tetracyclines and aminoglycosides results in effective treatment.

9.10   (b), (e)

Regulation of water secretion is by the distal tubule and the collecting ducts under the influence of vasopressin. The relative hyperosmolality of the medulla is maintained by a countercurrent mechanism and is responsible for the flux of water across the renal tubule.

9.11   (b), (e)

HCO$_3$ reabsorption (not secretion) is mediated at the proximal tubular level. Ammonia is secreted by the distal tubule. Sodium and glucose, as well as amino acids, are absorbed at the proximal tubule level.

9.12   (a), (b)
Growth hormone (GH) secretion occurs in a rhythmic fashion under the alternating influence of GHRH and somatostatin. This peaks in sleep. Insulin-like growth factor-1 (IGF-1) is a product of GH metabolism in the liver and is therefore not a direct regulator of GH levels in blood.

9.13   (a), (b), (c), (d)

9.14   (d), (e)
Dermatitis herpetiformis is associated with coeliac disease, axillary freckling with NF (neurofibromatosis), and periungual fibroma with tuberous sclerosis. Vitiligo is an autoimmune disorder and is closely related to many other similar disorders like Addison's disease, insulin-dependent diabetes mellitus (IDDM) and alopecia areata.

9.15   (a), (c)
Potent triggers of renin secretion are low sodium states and low blood volume.

9.16   None
Renin by itself is not a vasoconstrictor. Angiotensin I is converted into the active form angiotensin II by angiotensin-converting enzyme; PGI_2 is prostacyclin, which is a vasodilator.

9.17   (a), (e)

9.18   (b), (d), (e)
Hand, foot and mouth disease is an infection caused by Coxsackie virus presenting in young children with red, vesicular lesions on the palms, soles and in the oral cavity. It is self-limiting and carries a good prognosis. Parvovirus B19 causes aplastic crises in many haemolytic disorders, including sickle cell anaemia and spherocytosis. This results from its action on suppressing bone marrow precursors.

9.19   (a), (b), (c), (e)

9.20   (b), (d)
Causes for a high TSH in a neonate are transient hypothyroidism of the newborn, thyroid agenesis, thyroid enzyme defects and rarely maternal

drug intake. Maternal Graves' disease leads to a low thyroid stimulating hormone in the infant. Severe maternal iodine deficiency can cause neonatal hypothyroidism and high TSH, although it is quite rare.

9.21   (c), (d)

In anaemia of chronic inflammation, there is a normocytic, normo-chromic picture on the blood film. Serum iron and transferrin are low, but ferritin is normal. Impairment of iron utilisation occurs rather than true deficiency. Treatment of the underlying chronic disorder results in correction of the anaemia.

9.22   (b), (c), (d)

Unconjugated bilirubin is elevated in haemolysis and reduces levels of haptoglobulin (a bilirubin binding protein in the serum). Intravascular haemolysis causes leakage of haemoglobin into the urine and causes haemosiderinuria in the renal tubular cells. Polychromasia is a reflection of high reticulocyte count. Relative deficiency of folate occurs due to high demand and causes a megaloblastic marrow picture.

9.23   (b)

There are no discernible P waves in ventricular tachycardia. QRS duration is prolonged and bizarre QRS complexes are seen. It is a complication of untreated hyperthyroidism. The treatment of choice includes lignocaine and DC shock. Synchronised DC shock and adenosine are used in SVT (supraventricular tachycardia).

9.24   (a), (b), (c), (d), (e)

Pale stools and cough would mean cystic fibrosis, *Aspergillus* precipitin suggests allergic aspergillosis, calcified nodes indicate sarcoidosis, dextrocardia suggests Kartagener's syndrome and whooping cough in the past suggests an underlying bronchiectasis.

9.25   (c), (e)

DLCO is diffusion capacity for CO and is decreased in any condition that decreases effective alveolar surface area or affects the alveolar membrane. Examples include emphysema in which alveolar surface area is reduced, and pulmonary fibrosis in which there is reduced alveolar transfer of CO.

9.26   (a), (b), (d)

Antithrombin III is produced by the liver and acts as the main physiological inhibitor of coagulation. It is also a cofactor for heparin therapy. Congenital deficiency is familial and presents with thrombosis in the teenage group. Protein C is an important regulatory protein and inactivates factors Va and VIIIa. In heterozygotes, the protein level reaches 50% of normal and thromboembolic disease is common. Homozygotes die of purpura fulminans in infancy.

9.27   (d)

21-hydroxylase deficiency is the commonest form of CAH, and presents in two-thirds of cases as the classical salt-losing type, with virilisation due to the excess steroids produced proximal to the defect. The genes for this condition have been localised to the short arm of chromosome 6. There is autosomal recessive transmittance. Prenatal diagnosis is possible using DNA probes for the affected gene. 17-OH progesterone levels are elevated in amniotic fluid. Hypertension is a sign found in 11-hydroxylase deficiency, due to the excess deoxycortisol produced prior to the defect.

9.28   (b), (c)

Cisapride is a prokinetic drug that reduces gastric emptying time. It is not licensed for use in children in the UK. QT abnormalities are reported with therapy especially when given with erythromycin or antifungal drugs like ketoconazole (enzyme inhibitor) and have caused fatal arrythmias. This is especially common in children with a prolonged QT syndrome.

9.29   (b), (c)

9.30   (d), (e)

Nocturnal enuresis is commonly defined as persistence of enuresis beyond 4 years. Secondary causes include diabetes insipidus, diabetes mellitus, UTI, transient emotional stress, sexual abuse and neurological problems of bladder control. An interval of at least 6 months or more should elapse between toilet control being attained and return of enuretic symptoms to term it pathological.

Section 10

10.1 (a), (d)
Cri-du-chat syndrome is the result of a deletion in the short arm of chromosome 5. Infants with this syndrome have a characteristic cry due to the floppy larynx, resembling a cat's cry. Marfan's and homocystinuria are phenotypically similar but have different modes of inheritance (autosomal dominant vs. autosomal recessive). Kearns–Sayre syndrome is transmitted by mitochondrial DNA; it consists of progressive ophthalmoplegia and myopathy with lactic acidosis.

10.2 (b), (c), (d), (e)
Mutations in the fibrillin 1 gene are seen with Marfan's syndrome. This protein is a structural component of many microfibrils. There are 10 types of Ehlers–Danlos syndrome, each with characteristic features and individual gene mutations in procollagen or collagen. The syndrome presents due to a deficiency of collagen. Hypermobile joints, hyper-extensible skin, easy scarring and gaping wounds are common. Keratoconus and corneal scarring are common in some types.

10.3 (a), (c), (e)
These foramina form part of the ventricular system and its commun-ication with the subarachnoid system. The foramen of Monro lies between the anterior horns of the lateral ventricles and the midline, foramen of Magendie and Luschka are between the IV ventricle and the subarachnoid space. The other two foramina are seen in the skull base (foramen ovale transmits the mandibular component of the V nerve).

10.4 (a), (c)
In myotonic dystrophy, an affected mother may have very few symptoms (e.g. myotonia when hand is shaken) but the affected infant has severe muscle weakness and may need ventilation in the neonatal period. Frontal baldness, testicular atrophy and cataracts are common in affected males. This condition represents a classical example of genetic anticipa-tion.

10.5 (b), (c)
Recurrent meningococcal infection should prompt a search for a complement deficiency, especially in the terminal part of the cascade, C5 to C9. Recurrent staphylococcal infections are a presenting feature in chronic granulomatous disease (deficient intracellular killing), *Pneumocystis carinii* (PCP) is commonly found in cell-mediated immune deficiency (e.g. Di George syndrome) and delayed separation of the cord is seen with leucocyte adhesion deficiency.

10.6 (b), (d)
Acetazolamide is an inhibitor of carbonic anhydrase. It is used in post-hemorrhagic hydrocephalus (often with frusemide) and in reducing intra-ocular pressure. However, a recent multicentre trial has not supported the use of acetazolamide in preventing progression of post-haemorrhagic hydrocephalus. It causes metabolic acidosis due to the HCO_3^- loss in the renal tubule and thus also causes low K^+, just as in renal tubular acidosis.

10.7 (a), (d)
Note the double negative in choice (a).

10.8 (b), (e)
Sodium valproate is used in almost all seizure types except in infantile spasms (drugs of choice include nitrazepam, ACTH and prednisolone) and status epilepticus (drugs of choice include lorazepam, diazepam and midazolam). It is usually safe except for its hepatotoxicity and the association of a Reye-like syndrome.

10.9 (a), (b), (c)
Legionella pneumonia is a serious form of infection in the immuno-compromised patient. It classically presents with a diffuse pneumonia, hyponatraemia, diarrhoea, uraemia and a high phosphate level. Treatment is with erythromycin. Q fever is caused by *Coxiella burnetti* and presents in a normal host with an atypical pneumonia and is not associated with a rash. The main complication is an endocarditis in children with a previous heart disease. Treatment is with tetracycline or chloramphenicol.

10.10   (a), (d), (e)

Saccharin, fat chance! Desmin, vimentin are primitive muscle proteins; dystrophin is deficient in Becker and Duchenne muscular dystrophy. Keratin is not a muscle protein.

10.11 (c)

A diagnosis of CF is made on two positive sweat test results: Na > 60 mmol/l, Cl > 60 mmol/l (minimum amount of sweat = 100 mg), with clinical features. Genetic study to identify the commonest mutation in Caucasians in the ΔF-508 gene is diagnostic when it is homozygous. A combination of this mutation and a different one on the other chromosome is still diagnostic of CF. So far, around 400 mutations have been implicated in the causation of CF.

10.12 (a), (b), (d), (e)

Presenting features of gastro-oesophageal reflux (GER) in infants include all these other than the obvious symptom of vomiting. Persistent crying may be due to reflux oesophagitis from acid reflux. Recurrent cough and wheezing, persistent and recurrent pneumonias and recurrent cyanotic episodes are other presenting features.

10.13   (a), (c)

10.14   (a), (b), (d)

Candida infection of the nappy area is distinguished from seborrhoea by the fact that the latter does not involve the creases. Treatment of seborrhoeic dermatitis is with keratolytics such as salicylic acid derivatives, selenium compounds for the scalp, and topical steroids.

10.15 (a), (b), (d), (e)

Growth hormone (GH) secretion occurs in a rhythmic fashion under the alternating influence of GHRH and somatostatin. This peaks in sleep. Insulin-like growth factor-2 (IGF-2) is a product of GH metabolism in the liver and is therefore not a direct regulator of GH levels in blood. Hypoglycaemia is a potent stimulus for secretion of GH, being the basis for an insulin tolerance test for testing GH stimulation.

10.16 (b), (d)

Henoch–Schoenlein purpura and Kawasaki disease are the two commonest vasculitic illnesses in children. SLE is uncommon. Polyarteritis nodosa is an auto-immune vasculitis affecting middle-aged males; renal involvement is the most serious complication. The Churg–Strauss variant is highly related to an atopic individual; asthma is prominent as a presenting feature. Skin vasculitis and renal involvement follow. Prognosis is good with steroid therapy. Many cases of this syndrome have been reported in patients on zafirlucast (leukotriene antagonist used in asthma).

10.17 (c), (e)

Hypoglycaemia and low serum sodium are initial problems with TPN, not a long-term complication. Inadequate phosphate and calcium in TPN for premature infants leads to metabolic bone disease of prematurity, with high serum alkaline phosphatase and low phosphate, as well as changes of rickets on X-rays.

10.18 (a), (d)

Systemic *Aspergillus* infection is a serious complication of immuno-suppression and presents as a cerebral abscess, endocarditis, sinopul-monary infections, invasive otitis and endophthalmitis. *Candida* hyphae are seen on KOH preparations of affected sites. Molluscum contagiosum is a viral disease caused by a pox virus. Mucormycosis is seen in debilitated diabetics, usually adults with poor control and immunosuppression. *Microsporum* is transmitted from dogs and causes hair and scalp infection in humans (*Tinea capitis*).

10.19 (a), (b), (c), (d)

Choice (e) may cause secondary diabetes, not type I diabetes. DIDMOAD is DI (diabetes insipidus), DM (diabetes mellitus), OA (optic atrophy) and D (deafness). Type I polyglandular disease consists of Addison's disease, hypoparathyroidism and mucocutaneous candidiasis. Other autoimmune conditions such as alopecia arealis, pernicious anaemia, gonadal failure, CAH, IDDM and vitiligo may also occur at varying times. Type II (also called Schmidt syndrome) comprises IDDM, auto-immune thyroid disease and Addison disease.

10.20 (a), (b), (e)

Apnoea of prematurity is common in premature babies under 32 weeks gestation. This is possibly due to a poorly developed respiratory centre, poor chemoreceptor response to hypercarbia and hypoxia and poor respiratory muscle function. Theophylline was used as a modality of treatment, but due to a narrow therapeutic window and the necessity to monitor serum levels, it has been replaced by caffeine as drug of choice. Doxapram may be used as second line agent. In extreme cases, ventilation may be needed.

10.21 (b), (c), (d), (e)

Fanconi anaemia is a cause of aplastic anaemia, not Fanconi syndrome (characterised by renal tubular leak of phosphate, glucose and amino acids, and associated with proximal renal tubular acidosis).

10.22 (a), (c)

10.23 (a), (c), (d), (e)

PR interval prolongation > 0.20 s is abnormal at any age. A right axis is common in the first 3–4 years of life and this changes to normal axis by 6–7 years of age. Corrected QT interval (QT/square root RR interval) is usually < 0.45 s. T-wave inversion in the V1 and V2 leads may be normal upto 6 years and also sometimes upto 15 or 16 years. P-wave voltage > 2.5 mV indicates right atrial hypertrophy.

10.24 (a), (b), (d), (e)

Short stature (Turner syndrome), weight loss and abdominal pain (Crohn's disease), lanugo hair and low temperature (anorexia nervosa) and a family history (constitutional delay, which may be associated with short stature and a delayed bone age) may be clues to a diagnosis. Multiple large café-au-lait spots are clues to McCune–Albright syndrome and associated precocious puberty in girls.

10.25 (a), (b)

This is an indicator of small airways disease. In kyphoscoliosis, a restrictive pattern of lung function tests is seen with a low FEV_1 and low FVC, normal ratio of FEV_1/FVC. Croup is a result of upper airway obstruction due to inflammation in the trachea, larynx and bronchi.

10.26 (a), (c)
In assessing a child with suspected non-accidental injury, it is essential to know the normal development of the child's age group. Masturbation is common in the preschool age group. Bruising in areas of recurrent trauma is common in toddlers and preschool-, as well as school-age, children.

10.27 (c), (e)
Infantile autism presents usually before 30 months of age with poor social interaction, impaired verbal and non-verbal communication and poor imaginative activity. A strong genetic component has been identified - there is 80% concordance in monozygotic twins. No specific biochemical abnormalities have been identified and no drug treatment is of consistent benefit. Tantrums are common when the child's routine is upset.

10.28 (b)
Haemolytic anaemia is a result of cold agglutinins, which cause intravascular haemolysis. These are readily manifested on the blood film as rouleaux formation. All the other choices indicate rare complications.

10.29 (a), (b), (c), (d), (e)

10.30 (a), (b)
Cytochrome P450 enzymes are induced by phenobarbitone. Ceruloplasmin is not an enzyme, physostigmine antagonises anticholinesterase, and fluoride ions antagonise enolase (a step in glycolysis).

SCORING SHEETS

Section 1

	(a)	(b)	(c)	(d)	(e)	Score		(a)	(b)	(c)	(d)	(e)	Score
1.	☐	☐	☐	☐	☐	.....	16.	☐	☐	☐	☐	☐	.....
2.	☐	☐	☐	☐	☐	.....	17.	☐	☐	☐	☐	☐	.....
3.	☐	☐	☐	☐	☐	.....	18.	☐	☐	☐	☐	☐	.....
4.	☐	☐	☐	☐	☐	.....	19.	☐	☐	☐	☐	☐	.....
5.	☐	☐	☐	☐	☐	.....	20.	☐	☐	☐	☐	☐	.....
6.	☐	☐	☐	☐	☐	.....	21.	☐	☐	☐	☐	☐	.....
7.	☐	☐	☐	☐	☐	.....	22.	☐	☐	☐	☐	☐	.....
8.	☐	☐	☐	☐	☐	.....	23.	☐	☐	☐	☐	☐	.....
9.	☐	☐	☐	☐	☐	.....	24.	☐	☐	☐	☐	☐	.....
10.	☐	☐	☐	☐	☐	.....	25.	☐	☐	☐	☐	☐	.....
11.	☐	☐	☐	☐	☐	.....	26.	☐	☐	☐	☐	☐	.....
12.	☐	☐	☐	☐	☐	.....	27.	☐	☐	☐	☐	☐	.....
13.	☐	☐	☐	☐	☐	.....	28.	☐	☐	☐	☐	☐	.....
14.	☐	☐	☐	☐	☐	.....	29.	☐	☐	☐	☐	☐	.....
15.	☐	☐	☐	☐	☐	.....	30.	☐	☐	☐	☐	☐	.....

INSTRUCTIONS FOR SCORING:

1. Against each question, tick the appropriate choices. More than one choice (or none) may be correct.
2. Compare your answers with the correct answers.
3. Score yourself one mark for each correct response.
4. Your total score is out of a maximum possible score of 150.

SCORING SHEETS

Section 2

	(a)	(b)	(c)	(d)	(e)	Score		(a)	(b)	(c)	(d)	(e)	Score
1.	☐	☐	☐	☐	☐	.....	16.	☐	☐	☐	☐	☐	.....
2.	☐	☐	☐	☐	☐	.....	17.	☐	☐	☐	☐	☐	.....
3.	☐	☐	☐	☐	☐	.....	18.	☐	☐	☐	☐	☐	.....
4.	☐	☐	☐	☐	☐	.....	19.	☐	☐	☐	☐	☐	.....
5.	☐	☐	☐	☐	☐	.....	20.	☐	☐	☐	☐	☐	.....
6.	☐	☐	☐	☐	☐	.....	21.	☐	☐	☐	☐	☐	.....
7.	☐	☐	☐	☐	☐	.....	22.	☐	☐	☐	☐	☐	.....
8.	☐	☐	☐	☐	☐	.....	23.	☐	☐	☐	☐	☐	.....
9.	☐	☐	☐	☐	☐	.....	24.	☐	☐	☐	☐	☐	.....
10.	☐	☐	☐	☐	☐	.....	25.	☐	☐	☐	☐	☐	.....
11.	☐	☐	☐	☐	☐	.....	26.	☐	☐	☐	☐	☐	.....
12.	☐	☐	☐	☐	☐	.....	27.	☐	☐	☐	☐	☐	.....
13.	☐	☐	☐	☐	☐	.....	28.	☐	☐	☐	☐	☐	.....
14.	☐	☐	☐	☐	☐	.....	29.	☐	☐	☐	☐	☐	.....
15.	☐	☐	☐	☐	☐	.....	30.	☐	☐	☐	☐	☐	.....

INSTRUCTIONS FOR SCORING:

1. Against each question, tick the appropriate choices. More than one choice (or none) may be correct.
2. Compare your answers with the correct answers.
3. Score yourself one mark for each correct response.
4. Your total score is out of a maximum possible score of 150.

SCORING SHEETS

Section 3

	(a)	(b)	(c)	(d)	(e)	Score		(a)	(b)	(c)	(d)	(e)	Score
1.	☐	☐	☐	☐	☐	.....	16.	☐	☐	☐	☐	☐	.....
2.	☐	☐	☐	☐	☐	.....	17.	☐	☐	☐	☐	☐	.....
3.	☐	☐	☐	☐	☐	.....	18.	☐	☐	☐	☐	☐	.....
4.	☐	☐	☐	☐	☐	.....	19.	☐	☐	☐	☐	☐	.....
5.	☐	☐	☐	☐	☐	.....	20.	☐	☐	☐	☐	☐	.....
6.	☐	☐	☐	☐	☐	.....	21.	☐	☐	☐	☐	☐	.....
7.	☐	☐	☐	☐	☐	.....	22.	☐	☐	☐	☐	☐	.....
8.	☐	☐	☐	☐	☐	.....	23.	☐	☐	☐	☐	☐	.....
9.	☐	☐	☐	☐	☐	.....	24.	☐	☐	☐	☐	☐	.....
10.	☐	☐	☐	☐	☐	.....	25.	☐	☐	☐	☐	☐	.....
11.	☐	☐	☐	☐	☐	.....	26.	☐	☐	☐	☐	☐	.....
12.	☐	☐	☐	☐	☐	.....	27.	☐	☐	☐	☐	☐	.....
13.	☐	☐	☐	☐	☐	.....	28.	☐	☐	☐	☐	☐	.....
14.	☐	☐	☐	☐	☐	.....	29.	☐	☐	☐	☐	☐	.....
15.	☐	☐	☐	☐	☐	.....	30.	☐	☐	☐	☐	☐	.....

INSTRUCTIONS FOR SCORING:

1. Against each question, tick the appropriate choices. More than one choice (or none) may be correct.
2. Compare your answers with the correct answers.
3. Score yourself one mark for each correct response.
4. Your total score is out of a maximum possible score of 150.

SCORING SHEETS

Section 4

	(a)	(b)	(c)	(d)	(e)	Score		(a)	(b)	(c)	(d)	(e)	Score
1.	☐	☐	☐	☐	☐	.....	16.	☐	☐	☐	☐	☐	.....
2.	☐	☐	☐	☐	☐	.....	17.	☐	☐	☐	☐	☐	.....
3.	☐	☐	☐	☐	☐	.....	18.	☐	☐	☐	☐	☐	.....
4.	☐	☐	☐	☐	☐	.....	19.	☐	☐	☐	☐	☐	.....
5.	☐	☐	☐	☐	☐	.....	20.	☐	☐	☐	☐	☐	.....
6.	☐	☐	☐	☐	☐	.....	21.	☐	☐	☐	☐	☐	.....
7.	☐	☐	☐	☐	☐	.....	22.	☐	☐	☐	☐	☐	.....
8.	☐	☐	☐	☐	☐	.....	23.	☐	☐	☐	☐	☐	.....
9.	☐	☐	☐	☐	☐	.....	24.	☐	☐	☐	☐	☐	.....
10.	☐	☐	☐	☐	☐	.....	25.	☐	☐	☐	☐	☐	.....
11.	☐	☐	☐	☐	☐	.....	26.	☐	☐	☐	☐	☐	.....
12.	☐	☐	☐	☐	☐	.....	27.	☐	☐	☐	☐	☐	.....
13.	☐	☐	☐	☐	☐	.....	28.	☐	☐	☐	☐	☐	.....
14.	☐	☐	☐	☐	☐	.....	29.	☐	☐	☐	☐	☐	.....
15.	☐	☐	☐	☐	☐	.....	30.	☐	☐	☐	☐	☐	.....

INSTRUCTIONS FOR SCORING:

1. Against each question, tick the appropriate choices. More than one choice (or none) may be correct.
2. Compare your answers with the correct answers.
3. Score yourself one mark for each correct response.
4. Your total score is out of a maximum possible score of 150.

SCORING SHEETS

Section 5

	(a)	(b)	(c)	(d)	(e)	Score		(a)	(b)	(c)	(d)	(e)	Score
1.	☐	☐	☐	☐	☐	.....	16.	☐	☐	☐	☐	☐	.....
2.	☐	☐	☐	☐	☐	.....	17.	☐	☐	☐	☐	☐	.....
3.	☐	☐	☐	☐	☐	.....	18.	☐	☐	☐	☐	☐	.....
4.	☐	☐	☐	☐	☐	.....	19.	☐	☐	☐	☐	☐	.....
5.	☐	☐	☐	☐	☐	.....	20.	☐	☐	☐	☐	☐	.....
6.	☐	☐	☐	☐	☐	.....	21.	☐	☐	☐	☐	☐	.....
7.	☐	☐	☐	☐	☐	.....	22.	☐	☐	☐	☐	☐	.....
8.	☐	☐	☐	☐	☐	.....	23.	☐	☐	☐	☐	☐	.....
9.	☐	☐	☐	☐	☐	.....	24.	☐	☐	☐	☐	☐	.....
10.	☐	☐	☐	☐	☐	.....	25.	☐	☐	☐	☐	☐	.....
11.	☐	☐	☐	☐	☐	.....	26.	☐	☐	☐	☐	☐	.....
12.	☐	☐	☐	☐	☐	.....	27.	☐	☐	☐	☐	☐	.....
13.	☐	☐	☐	☐	☐	.....	28.	☐	☐	☐	☐	☐	.....
14.	☐	☐	☐	☐	☐	.....	29.	☐	☐	☐	☐	☐	.....
15.	☐	☐	☐	☐	☐	.....	30.	☐	☐	☐	☐	☐	.....

INSTRUCTIONS FOR SCORING:

1. Against each question, tick the appropriate choices. More than one choice (or none) may be correct.
2. Compare your answers with the correct answers.
3. Score yourself one mark for each correct response.
4. Your total score is out of a maximum possible score of 150.

SCORING SHEETS

Section 6

	(a)	(b)	(c)	(d)	(e)	Score		(a)	(b)	(c)	(d)	(e)	Score
1.	☐	☐	☐	☐	☐	.....	16.	☐	☐	☐	☐	☐	.....
2.	☐	☐	☐	☐	☐	.....	17.	☐	☐	☐	☐	☐	.....
3.	☐	☐	☐	☐	☐	.....	18.	☐	☐	☐	☐	☐	.....
4.	☐	☐	☐	☐	☐	.....	19.	☐	☐	☐	☐	☐	.....
5.	☐	☐	☐	☐	☐	.....	20.	☐	☐	☐	☐	☐	.....
6.	☐	☐	☐	☐	☐	.....	21.	☐	☐	☐	☐	☐	.....
7.	☐	☐	☐	☐	☐	.....	22.	☐	☐	☐	☐	☐	.....
8.	☐	☐	☐	☐	☐	.....	23.	☐	☐	☐	☐	☐	.....
9.	☐	☐	☐	☐	☐	.....	24.	☐	☐	☐	☐	☐	.....
10.	☐	☐	☐	☐	☐	.....	25.	☐	☐	☐	☐	☐	.....
11.	☐	☐	☐	☐	☐	.....	26.	☐	☐	☐	☐	☐	.....
12.	☐	☐	☐	☐	☐	.....	27.	☐	☐	☐	☐	☐	.....
13.	☐	☐	☐	☐	☐	.....	28.	☐	☐	☐	☐	☐	.....
14.	☐	☐	☐	☐	☐	.....	29.	☐	☐	☐	☐	☐	.....
15.	☐	☐	☐	☐	☐	.....	30.	☐	☐	☐	☐	☐	.....

INSTRUCTIONS FOR SCORING:

1. Against each question, tick the appropriate choices. More than one choice (or none) may be correct.
2. Compare your answers with the correct answers.
3. Score yourself one mark for each correct response.
4. Your total score is out of a maximum possible score of 150.

<u>SCORING SHEETS</u>

Section 7

	(a)	(b)	(c)	(d)	(e)	Score		(a)	(b)	(c)	(d)	(e)	Score
1.	☐	☐	☐	☐	☐	.....	16.	☐	☐	☐	☐	☐	.....
2.	☐	☐	☐	☐	☐	.....	17.	☐	☐	☐	☐	☐	.....
3.	☐	☐	☐	☐	☐	.....	18.	☐	☐	☐	☐	☐	.....
4.	☐	☐	☐	☐	☐	.....	19.	☐	☐	☐	☐	☐	.....
5.	☐	☐	☐	☐	☐	.....	20.	☐	☐	☐	☐	☐	.....
6.	☐	☐	☐	☐	☐	.....	21.	☐	☐	☐	☐	☐	.....
7.	☐	☐	☐	☐	☐	.....	22.	☐	☐	☐	☐	☐	.....
8.	☐	☐	☐	☐	☐	.....	23.	☐	☐	☐	☐	☐	.....
9.	☐	☐	☐	☐	☐	.....	24.	☐	☐	☐	☐	☐	.....
10.	☐	☐	☐	☐	☐	.....	25.	☐	☐	☐	☐	☐	.....
11.	☐	☐	☐	☐	☐	.....	26.	☐	☐	☐	☐	☐	.....
12.	☐	☐	☐	☐	☐	.....	27.	☐	☐	☐	☐	☐	.....
13.	☐	☐	☐	☐	☐	.....	28.	☐	☐	☐	☐	☐	.....
14.	☐	☐	☐	☐	☐	.....	29.	☐	☐	☐	☐	☐	.....
15.	☐	☐	☐	☐	☐	.....	30.	☐	☐	☐	☐	☐	.....

INSTRUCTIONS FOR SCORING:

1. Against each question, tick the appropriate choices. More than one choice (or none) may be correct.
2. Compare your answers with the correct answers.
3. Score yourself one mark for each correct response.
4. Your total score is out of a maximum possible score of 150.

SCORING SHEETS

Section 8

	(a)	(b)	(c)	(d)	(e)	Score		(a)	(b)	(c)	(d)	(e)	Score
1.	☐	☐	☐	☐	☐	.....	16.	☐	☐	☐	☐	☐	.....
2.	☐	☐	☐	☐	☐	.....	17.	☐	☐	☐	☐	☐	.....
3.	☐	☐	☐	☐	☐	.....	18.	☐	☐	☐	☐	☐	.....
4.	☐	☐	☐	☐	☐	.....	19.	☐	☐	☐	☐	☐	.....
5.	☐	☐	☐	☐	☐	.....	20.	☐	☐	☐	☐	☐	.....
6.	☐	☐	☐	☐	☐	.....	21.	☐	☐	☐	☐	☐	.....
7.	☐	☐	☐	☐	☐	.....	22.	☐	☐	☐	☐	☐	.....
8.	☐	☐	☐	☐	☐	.....	23.	☐	☐	☐	☐	☐	.....
9.	☐	☐	☐	☐	☐	.....	24.	☐	☐	☐	☐	☐	.....
10.	☐	☐	☐	☐	☐	.....	25.	☐	☐	☐	☐	☐	.....
11.	☐	☐	☐	☐	☐	.....	26.	☐	☐	☐	☐	☐	.....
12.	☐	☐	☐	☐	☐	.....	27.	☐	☐	☐	☐	☐	.....
13.	☐	☐	☐	☐	☐	.....	28.	☐	☐	☐	☐	☐	.....
14.	☐	☐	☐	☐	☐	.....	29.	☐	☐	☐	☐	☐	.....
15.	☐	☐	☐	☐	☐	.....	30.	☐	☐	☐	☐	☐	.....

INSTRUCTIONS FOR SCORING:

1. Against each question, tick the appropriate choices. More than one choice (or none) may be correct.
2. Compare your answers with the correct answers.
3. Score yourself one mark for each correct response.
4. Your total score is out of a maximum possible score of 150.

SCORING SHEETS

Section 9

	(a)	(b)	(c)	(d)	(e)	Score		(a)	(b)	(c)	(d)	(e)	Score
1.	☐	☐	☐	☐	☐	.....	16.	☐	☐	☐	☐	☐	.....
2.	☐	☐	☐	☐	☐	.....	17.	☐	☐	☐	☐	☐	.....
3.	☐	☐	☐	☐	☐	.....	18.	☐	☐	☐	☐	☐	.....
4.	☐	☐	☐	☐	☐	.....	19.	☐	☐	☐	☐	☐	.....
5.	☐	☐	☐	☐	☐	.....	20.	☐	☐	☐	☐	☐	.....
6.	☐	☐	☐	☐	☐	.....	21.	☐	☐	☐	☐	☐	.....
7.	☐	☐	☐	☐	☐	.....	22.	☐	☐	☐	☐	☐	.....
8.	☐	☐	☐	☐	☐	.....	23.	☐	☐	☐	☐	☐	.....
9.	☐	☐	☐	☐	☐	.....	24.	☐	☐	☐	☐	☐	.....
10.	☐	☐	☐	☐	☐	.....	25.	☐	☐	☐	☐	☐	.....
11.	☐	☐	☐	☐	☐	.....	26.	☐	☐	☐	☐	☐	.....
12.	☐	☐	☐	☐	☐	.....	27.	☐	☐	☐	☐	☐	.....
13.	☐	☐	☐	☐	☐	.....	28.	☐	☐	☐	☐	☐	.....
14.	☐	☐	☐	☐	☐	.....	29.	☐	☐	☐	☐	☐	.....
15.	☐	☐	☐	☐	☐	.....	30.	☐	☐	☐	☐	☐	.....

INSTRUCTIONS FOR SCORING:

1. Against each question, tick the appropriate choices. More than one choice (or none) may be correct.
2. Compare your answers with the correct answers.
3. Score yourself one mark for each correct response.
4. Your total score is out of a maximum possible score of 150.

SCORING SHEETS

Section 10

	(a)	(b)	(c)	(d)	(e)	Score		(a)	(b)	(c)	(d)	(e)	Score
1.	☐	☐	☐	☐	☐	.....	16.	☐	☐	☐	☐	☐	.....
2.	☐	☐	☐	☐	☐	.....	17.	☐	☐	☐	☐	☐	.....
3.	☐	☐	☐	☐	☐	.....	18.	☐	☐	☐	☐	☐	.....
4.	☐	☐	☐	☐	☐	.....	19.	☐	☐	☐	☐	☐	.....
5.	☐	☐	☐	☐	☐	.....	20.	☐	☐	☐	☐	☐	.....
6.	☐	☐	☐	☐	☐	.....	21.	☐	☐	☐	☐	☐	.....
7.	☐	☐	☐	☐	☐	.....	22.	☐	☐	☐	☐	☐	.....
8.	☐	☐	☐	☐	☐	.....	23.	☐	☐	☐	☐	☐	.....
9.	☐	☐	☐	☐	☐	.....	24.	☐	☐	☐	☐	☐	.....
10.	☐	☐	☐	☐	☐	.....	25.	☐	☐	☐	☐	☐	.....
11.	☐	☐	☐	☐	☐	.....	26.	☐	☐	☐	☐	☐	.....
12.	☐	☐	☐	☐	☐	.....	27.	☐	☐	☐	☐	☐	.....
13.	☐	☐	☐	☐	☐	.....	28.	☐	☐	☐	☐	☐	.....
14.	☐	☐	☐	☐	☐	.....	29.	☐	☐	☐	☐	☐	.....
15.	☐	☐	☐	☐	☐	.....	30.	☐	☐	☐	☐	☐	.....

INSTRUCTIONS FOR SCORING:

1. Against each question, tick the appropriate choices. More than one choice (or none) may be correct.
2. Compare your answers with the correct answers.
3. Score yourself one mark for each correct response.
4. Your total score is out of a maximum possible score of 150.

NOTES

NOTES

NOTES

NOTES

NOTES

NOTES